Computed-Tomography (CT) Scan

Edited by Reda R. Gharieb

Published in London, United Kingdom

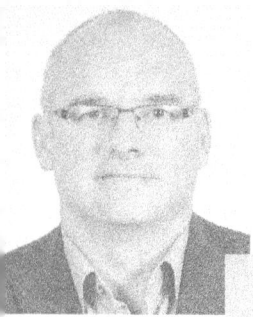
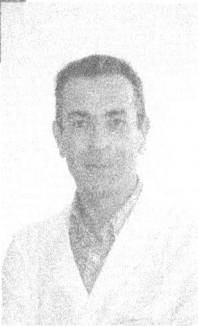
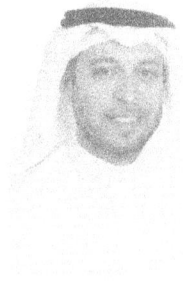
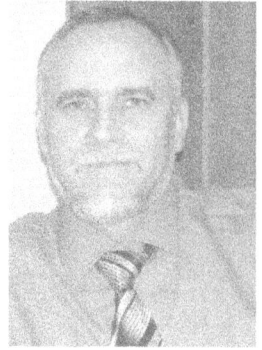
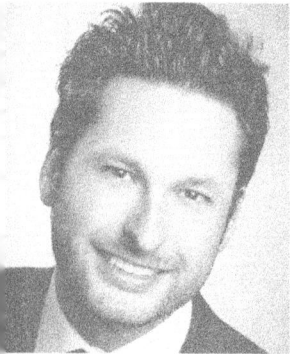
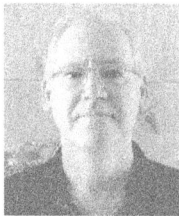
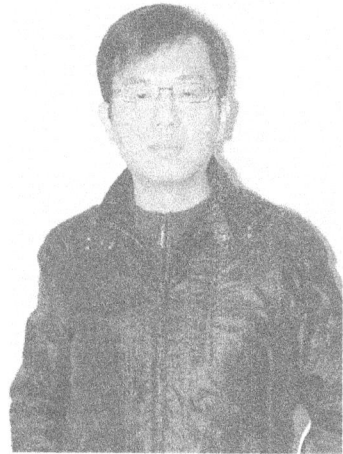

IntechOpen

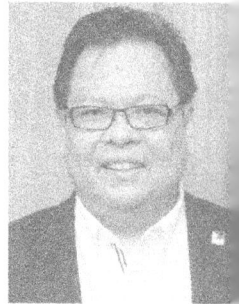
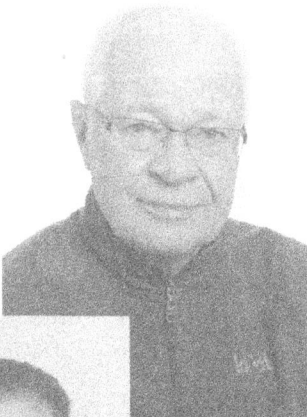
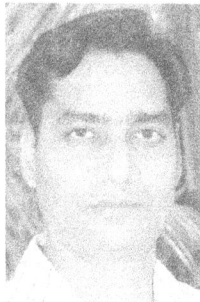
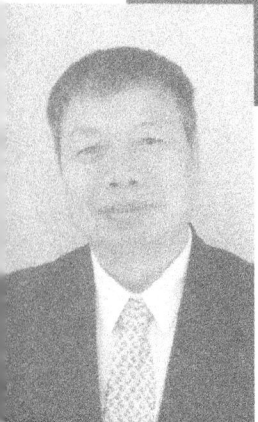
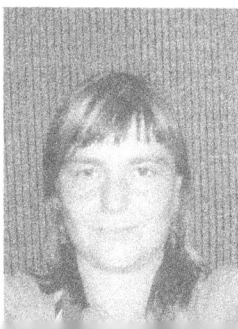
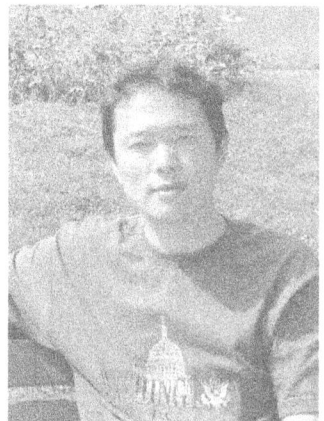

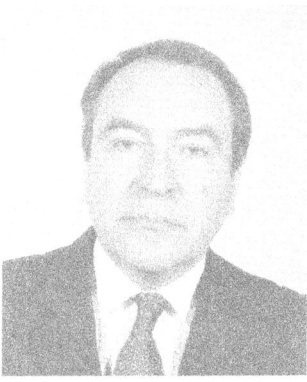

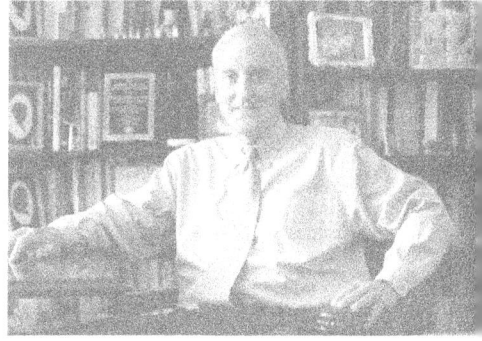

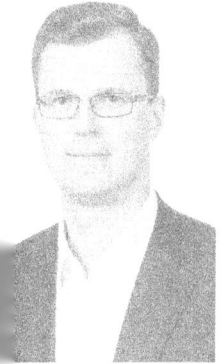

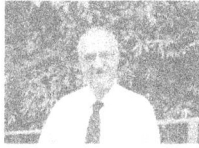

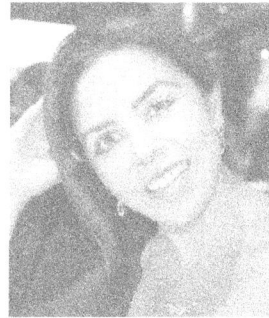

Supporting open minds since 2005

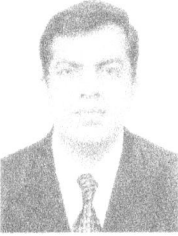

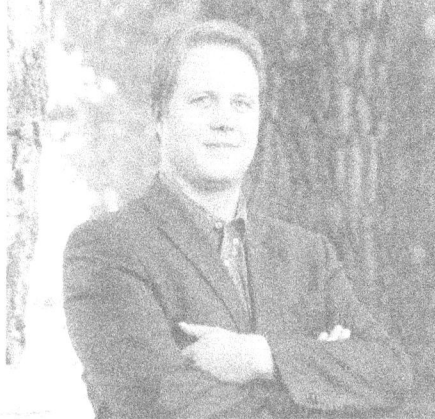

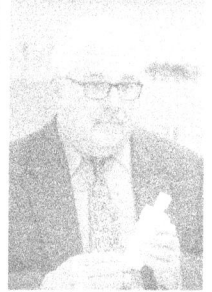

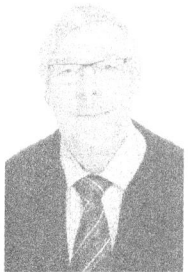

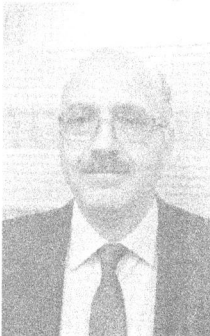

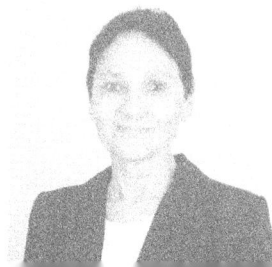

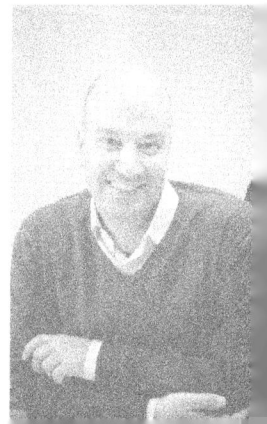

Computed-Tomography (CT) Scan
http://dx.doi.org/10.5772/intechopen.95180
Edited by Reda R. Gharieb

Contributors
Ivan Vasilievich Ivanov, Elena Ivanovna Matkevich, Sikandar Shaikh, Ibrahima Niang, Géraud Akpo, Khadidiatou Ndiaye Diouf, Sokhna Ba, Anil K. Bharodiya, Reda R. Gharieb

Notice
Statements and opinions expressed in the chapters are these of the individual contributors and not necessarily those of the editors or publisher. No responsibility is accepted for the accuracy of information contained in the published chapters. The publisher assumes no responsibility for any damage or injury to persons or property arising out of the use of any materials, instructions, methods or ideas contained in the book.

First published in London, United Kingdom, 2022 by IntechOpen
IntechOpen is the global imprint of INTECHOPEN LIMITED, registered in England and Wales, registration number: 11086078, 5 Princes Gate Court, London, SW7 2QJ, United Kingdom
Printed in Croatia

British Library Cataloguing-in-Publication Data
A catalogue record for this book is available from the British Library

Additional hard and PDF copies can be obtained from orders@intechopen.com

Computed-Tomography (CT) Scan
Edited by Reda R. Gharieb
p. cm.
Print ISBN 978-1-80355-117-3
Online ISBN 978-1-80355-118-0
eBook (PDF) ISBN 978-1-80355-119-7

We are IntechOpen,
the world's leading publisher of
Open Access books
Built by scientists, for scientists

5,800+
Open access books available

142,000+
International authors and editors

180M+
Downloads

Our authors are among the

156
Countries delivered to

Top 1%
most cited scientists

12.2%
Contributors from top 500 universities

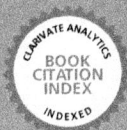

Interested in publishing with us?
Contact book.department@intechopen.com

Numbers displayed above are based on latest data collected.
For more information visit www.intechopen.com

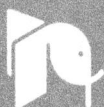

Meet the editor

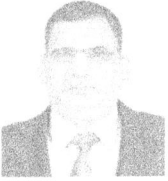

Reda R. Gharieb, Ph.D. is a Professor of Biomedical and Bioelectronics Engineering, Assiut University, Egypt. He served as a scientist in Japan and the United States. He worked for Fairway Medical Technologies Inc. and Seno Medical Instruments Inc., Texas, USA, on their photoacoustic imaging (PAI) technology. He developed algorithms for 2D image reconstruction in PAI of breast and prostate cancers. He also developed an algorithm for 3D image reconstruction in PAI of a small animal, using a rotated ARC-shaped sensor array. Dr. Gharieb has authored three books, four book chapters, two patents, and about sixty papers. He has also edited two books. His research interests include signal/image processing, modeling and simulation, statistical and scientific computing, bioinstrumentation, and computed tomography.

Contents

Preface

Computed tomography (CT) was introduced commercially for the first time by British engineer Godfrey Hounsfield in 1972. Since then, it has become the main imaging modality in hospitals and clinical centers. A CT scan can be used to visualize nearly all parts of the body to diagnose disease or injury as well as to plan medical, surgical, or radiation treatment. Particularly, it is well suited for quickly examining people who may have internal injuries from car accidents or other types of traumas. In addition, CT plays an important role in chest imaging in the current COVID-19 pandemic.

The book consists of five chapters. Chapter 1, by Dr. Reda R. Gharieb, presents the instrumentational basics of CT scanning, a mathematical and simulation review of a CT algorithm called the filtered back projection, in linear- and fan-beams projection, and some medical applications of CT imaging. Chapter 2, by Drs. Ibrahima Niang, Géraud Akpo, Khadidiatou Ndiaye Diouf, and Sokhna Ba, discusses the use of CT in the context of the coronavirus pandemic. It explains the effect of coronavirus on the lungs and how physicians can recognize this effect. Chapter 3, by Drs. Elena Ivanovna Matkevich and Ivan Vasilievich Ivanov presents a study of radiation doses and risk assessment during CT of the chest in COVID-19 patients. Chapter 4, by Dr. Sikandar Shaikh, presents the basics and applications of positron emission tomography (PET), an imaging technology that uses positron emission instead of X-rays. Finally, Chapter 5, by Dr. Anil K. Bharodiya, deals with handling, using different image processing methods, and final CT images for feature extraction in recognition of patterns.

The editor thanks the contributing authors for their efforts and for sharing their research. The editor also thanks and appreciates the service and support received from Author Service Managers Mrs. Dzeni Kalcic, Mrs. Nikolina Pomenic, and Mrs. Zrinka Tomicic at IntechOpen.

Finally, I hope that this book will be a useful resource for readers interested in advancing their knowledge and experience of CT scanning.

Reda R. Gharieb
Professor of Biomedical Engineering and Electronics,
Assiut University,
Assiut, Egypt

X-Rays and Computed Tomography Scan Imaging: Instrumentation and Medical Applications

Reda R. Gharieb

Abstract

This chapter gives a review for both conventional X-ray and computed tomography (CT) scan imaging modalities and their medical applications. The chapter presents a brief history on the discovery of X-ray, X-ray imaging, and computed tomography scan. The linear projection for the generation of the sinogram (the detector's signals versus the rotational angle) and the filtered backprojection for image reconstruction are discussed. Computer simulations for linear and fan beams X-ray are also presented. The chapter discusses some medical applications of both the conventional X-ray and CT scan imaging.

Keywords: X-ray tube, X-ray, bremsstrahlung, photons and electromagnetic waves, X-ray and dual x-ray imaging, CT scan imaging, linear projection, filtered backprojection, medical applications, chest, abdomen, bones, Covid-19

1. Introduction

In 1895, German physicist Wilhelm C. Roentgen accidentally noticed that a cathode-ray tube could make a sheet of paper coated with barium platinocyanide glow [1, 2]. This effect was even while the tube and the paper were in separate rooms. Roentgen decided that the tube must be emitting some sort of penetrating rays, which he named them X for unknown. Shortly afterward, Roentgen aimed the X-rays through Mrs. Roentgen's hand at a chemically coated screen. He could see the bones in the hand clearly on the screen. In 1905, Robert Kienböck, a German radiologist, could identify what named Kienböck's disease, using strips of silver bromide photographic paper to estimate the amount of radiation to which patients were exposed in radiation therapy [3–6]. Then, over the next few decades, X-rays grew into a widely used diagnostic tool. The image used to be captured on an X-ray-sensitive film. Technology advances of electronics made use of X-ray for digital imaging by replacing the traditional X-ray-sensitive film by electronic sensors [7–10]. Today, both convention and digital X-ray imaging modalities are the prompt and main diagnostic tools for investigating and screening the chest for viral and bacterial pneumonia, tuberculosis, lung cancer [11–19], enlarged heart, and blocked blood vessels [20–24]; the bones and teeth for fractures and infections, arthritis, bone cancer, and dental decay [25–30]; the abdomen for digestive tract problems and looking for swallowed items [31]. Moreover, other modalities for X-ray imaging have been developed such as digital mammography for breast cancer screening [32]. It is a special imaging technique that employs X-ray with low dose of energy. Dual-energy X-ray has also been developed and used for measuring bone mineral density (BMD) [33, 34]. In this technique, two different X-ray beams with different energy values are used.

The history of computed tomography (CT) scan has been around for almost 50 years. It was created by British engineer Godfrey Hounsfield of EMI Laboratories in 1972 [35], **Figure 1**. He co-invented the technology with physicist Dr. Allan Cormack. CT uses a computer algorithm to reconstruct an image from the intensity projections collected by detectors for all angles of rotation of both X-ray source and the detectors around the target; such an image is called a slice. Next slice is obtained after moving the target a step inside the gantry and repeating the rotation, collection, and reconstruct. This made it possible to detect diseases at the earliest stages. At the same time, the radiation load is minimal. Important advantages of CT scan are as follows: the possibility of obtaining three-dimensional images of internal organs, the speed of the performing, comfort of the patient. CT scan has been used for investigating and screening many organs and for different diseases [36–48]. Moreover, it could be used for brain imaging. For a CT scan slice, detectors acquire data versus rational angles, and the slice image is reconstructed by backprojection and filtered backprojection algorithms [49–55]. This chapter highlights instrumentation aspects and medical applications of conventional and CT scan X-ray technology.

2. X-ray and CT scan instruments

2.1 X-ray tube and generation of X-ray

X-ray tube consists of four main parts: the tube, the high-voltage generator, the control console, and the cooling system. The tube has a cathode filament heated by a small voltage providing a small current of few amps. When the filament is heated up, the electrons in the conduction wire start breaking free. To accelerate these electrons toward the anode, a strong electrical potential $(30 - 150)KV$ is maintained between the anode and the cathode. Electrons that break free of the cathode are

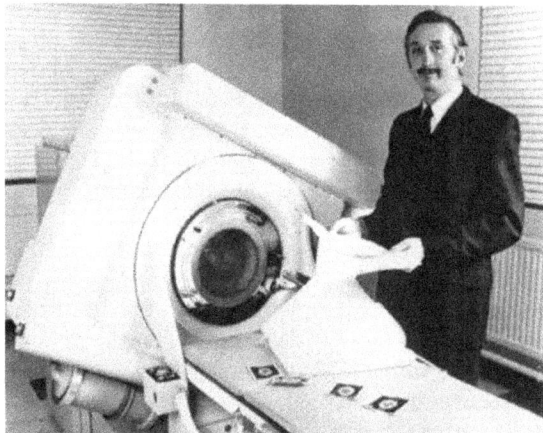

Figure 1.
Sir Godfrey Hounsfield with the first commercial CT scanner: http://www.edubilla.com/inventor/godfrey-hounsfield/.

strongly attracted to the anode disc. The electron flow between the cathode and the anode accounts for the tube current and is in the range of milliamps (mA). This current is controlled by regulating the filament current generated by the heating low voltage applied to the cathode circuit. The higher the temperature of the filament, the larger the number of electrons that leave the cathode and travel toward the anode. By controlling the filament temperature, the control console regulates the value of the filament current and hence the intensity of the X-ray output. **Figure 2** shows an illustrative X-ray tube, which consists of a vacuum glass with the node on one side and the cathode on the other side. The cathode, which is a filament being heated up, is the source of electrons. These electrons are accelerated by the applied high potential between the anode (positive terminal) and the cathode (negative terminal). The accelerated electrons, the electrons with high kinetic energy, bombarding the anode, penetrate the heavy-metal target, for example, tungsten, attached to the anode. Some of these electrons travel close to the nucleus of the heavy metal under the attraction force of its positive charge and are subsequently influenced by its electric field. Thus, these electrons would be deflected, and a portion or all of their kinetic energy would be lost. The principle of the conservation of energy states that in producing the X-ray photon, the electron has lost some of its kinetic energy (KE), which should be the energy of the X-ray photon. That is,

$$Final\ KE\ of\ electron = Initial\ KE\ of\ electron - Energy\ of\ X\_ray\ photon \qquad (1)$$

Thus, X-ray is an electromagnetic radiation (photons) of extremely short wavelength with wavelengths ranging from about 10^{-8} to $10^{-12} meter$ and corresponding very high frequencies from about 10^{16} to 10^{20} Hertz (Hz).

The energy of each photon is determined according to the plank's equation:

$$Energy\ of\ X\_ray\ photon = hf = \frac{hc}{\lambda} \qquad (2)$$

where $h = 4.14 \times 10^{-15} eVs$ is the Plank's constant, and $c = 3 \times 10^8 m/sec$ is the speed of light and λ is the wavelength in $meter$. **Figure 3** shows the Bremsstrahlung spectrum of tungsten X-ray. It is obvious that the maxim number of photons occurs at energy of 60 Kev. The photons of low energy are removed from the ray using filtering technique. Such filtering reduces the dose of low-energy photons exposing the patient.

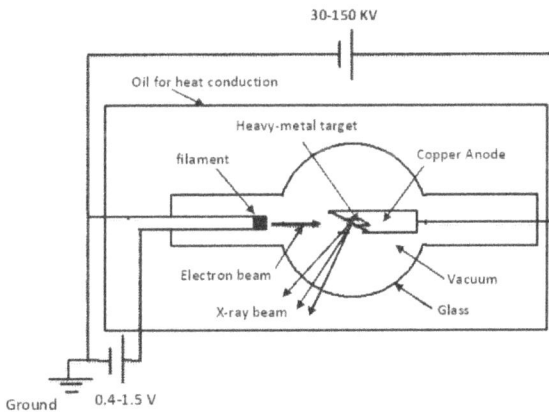

Figure 2.
X-ray tube.

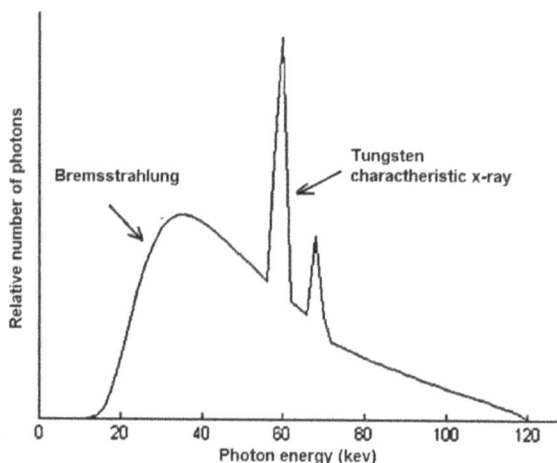

Figure 3.
Bremsstrahlung (brake spectrum) of tungsten.

1. X-ray imaging of human body

2. Non-digital imaging

When a human body is exposure to X-rays, the body soft tissue, such as the skin and organs, cannot absorb the high-energy rays, and the beam passes through them. However, dense tissues inside the human's bodies, such as bones, absorb the radiation. The amount of radiation passing through the tissue is detected on the other side by an X-ray-sensitive film for non-digital imaging. The film is made of gelatin-covered polyester base or cellulose base coated on one side or two sides by radio-sensitive emulsion, and the emulsion consists of silver halide crystals immersed in gelatin. The emulsion layer is sensitive to X-ray. After the exposure of the film to X-rays, it is processed to convert the latent image into visible one [56]. The film after being processed provides a grayscale image from black to white. The whiter a region of an X-ray image, the lesser the exposure of this region to X-ray and hence the denser the tissue corresponding to this image region. Bones and air show themselves, in an X-ray image, as white and black, respectively.

2.2 Digital X-ray imaging

In digital X-ray imaging, instead of using an X-ray-sensitive film to capture an image, a planar array of electronic sensors/detectors is used to capture the X-ray image [55]. Each electrical detector generates a signal, where its intensity is proportional to the number photons reached this detector. The output of the planar arrays can be displayed on a computer monitor as a grayscale image. These digital images can be stored on a hard drive and can be exchanged on the Internet between different clinical centers. There are two digital detection techniques, the first is called direct technique and the second is called indirect one:

2.2.1 Direct technique

Amorphous silicon (a-Si) or amorphous selenium (a-Se) is used to generate positive charges proportional to X-ray intensity [10, 55–57]. These positive charges

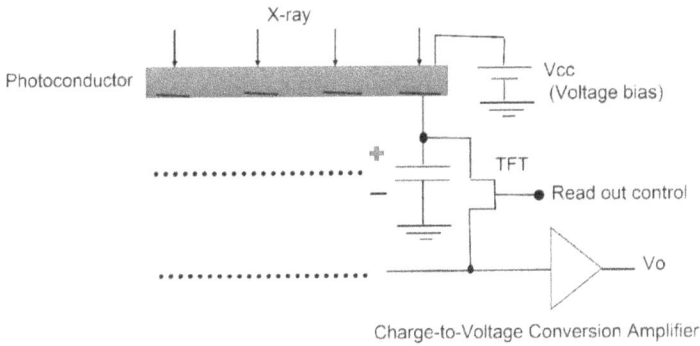

Figure 4.
Direct digital X-ray image capture. One pixel in a cross section of a linear array, all pixels in the array are similar. The readout control selects the pixel being readout. In a planar array, two readout controls are used for selecting the row and the column of the readout pixel. Advances in semiconductor electronics made it possible to fabricate a matrix of such single detector [10, 57].

are stored in capacitors until they are readout. The capacitor charge corresponding to each pixel is read using a thin flat transistor (TFT) and is converted to voltage, using a charge-to-voltage amplifier. **Figure 4** shows a single detector for one pixel. A matrix consisting of many single detectors can be fabricated similar to the one used in CCD (charge-coupled display).

2.2.2 Indirect technique

In this technique, the X-ray is first converted into visible light using an X-ray scintillator. Common materials used as scintillator are the gadolinium oxysulfide (GdO2S2) and cesium iodide (CsI) [10, 55–57]. A planar array of photodiodes, TFTs, and capacitors equal to the image size in pixels are used to detect the visible light. Each photodiode generates a current proportional to the intensity of light reached it, and this current is stored as a charge in the capacitor. The capacitor charge is read out using TFT and converted to voltage, using a charge-to-voltage conversion amplifier. **Figure 5** shows a detector element for one pixel.

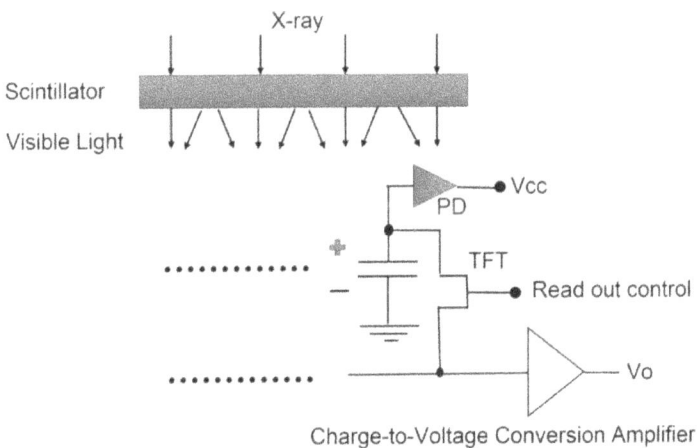

Figure 5.
Indirect digital X-ray image capture. One pixel in a cross section of a linear array, all pixels in the array or matrix are similar. The readout control signal selects the column and row of the pixel being readout.

3. CT scan imaging

3.1 CT scan machine

In conventional X-ray machine, one image of the body tissue is recorded by sending one beam of X-ray through the body from one side and detected attenuated X-ray beam from the body's other side. However, in CT scan machine, the patient lies on a table that moves through a doughnut-like ring known as a gantry. In each longitudinal position of the patient's table, a series of X-ray data are collected from different angles around the body. This is by enabling the X-ray tube and the X-ray detector array to rotate around the body. A computer algorithm is sued to generate an axial image called a slice from all X-ray data collected from all angles around the body position. Next slice is obtained by moving the patient's table through the gantry and repeating the rotation of X-ray tube and the detector array and collecting the X-ray data from all angles around the patient at this new position. **Figure 6** shows an illustrative sectional diagram for a CT scan machine.

3.2 Computed tomography (CT)

Computed tomography consists of two main steps. The first one is the acquisition of X-ray passing tissue, by different detectors from different angles around the target. This is carried out by shining X-ray beam on the target and detecting the amount of passed X-rays reached at each detector on the opposite side. This acquired data is mathematically explained by the theory of linear projection. The acquiring step provides the sinogram, which is the X-ray intensity at each detector versus rotational angles around the body. The second step is the reconstruction of the image from the acquired sinogram. This image reconstruction, the reverse process, is explained by the theory of backprojection.

3.2.1 Linear beam projection

In **Figure 7**, an X-ray passes through a target from the source to the detector on the line determined by the parameters: the distance, $-\infty \leq s \leq \infty$, in cm and the angle, $0 \leq \theta \leq \pi$, in degree. The intensity of this X -ray, at the detector, is given by

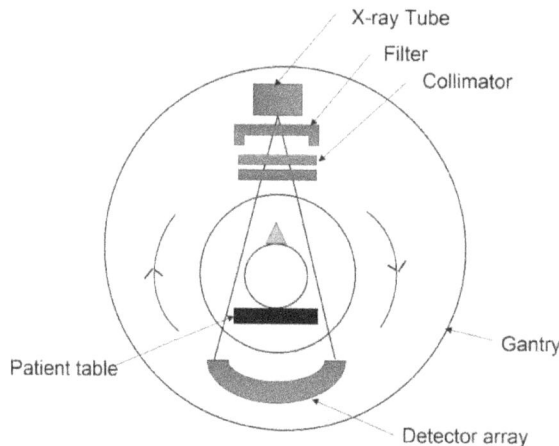

Figure 6.
An illustrative sectional diagram of a CT scan machine.

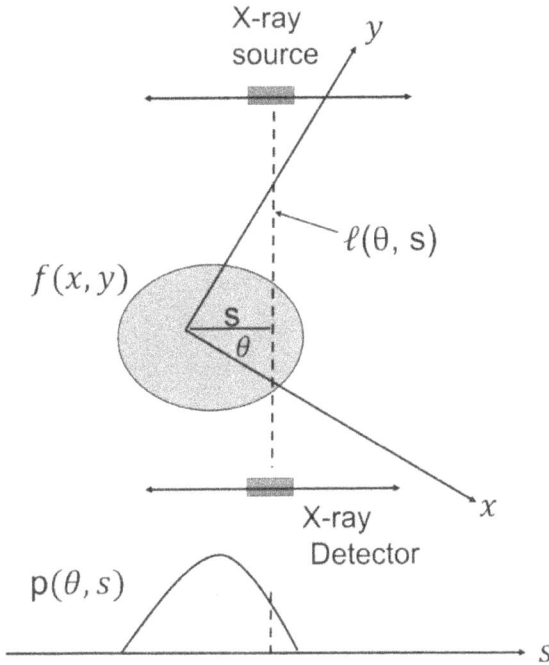

Figure 7.
An intensity function $f(x,y)$ and the linear projection $p(\theta,s)$ versus the distance s at certain angle $0 \leq \theta \leq \pi$.

$$I = I_0 e^{-\int_{\ell(\theta,s)} f(x,y)dxdy} \tag{3}$$

where I_0 is the intensity at the source. Simply to get the projection $\int_{\ell(\theta,s)} f(x,y)dxdy$, the logarithmic can be used

$$p(\theta,s) = \ln\left(\frac{I_0}{I}\right) = \int_{\ell(\theta,s)} f(x,y)dxdy \tag{4}$$

Notice that this logarithmic operation is implemented naturally by different detectors. Thus, the detected value $\ln\left(\frac{I_0}{I}\right)$ or the projection $p(\theta,s)$ is a linear integration of absorption coefficients of all voxels over the line $\ell(\theta,s)$. This line is parameterized by θ and s as follows

$$\ell(\theta,s) = \{(x,y) : x\cos(\theta) + y\sin(\theta) = s\} \tag{5}$$

Also Eq. (4) can be written as

$$p(\theta,s) = \int_x \int_y f((x,y)\delta(x\cos(\theta) + y\,\sin(\theta) - s)dxdy \tag{6}$$

where $\delta(0) = 1$.

It is obvious that due to the integration of the absorption coefficients of all voxels on the line $\ell(\theta,s)$, we lost the information about which voxels on the line have high or low absorption coefficients. **Figure 8(a)** shows a computer simulation scenario in which an intensity function has three objects with different absorption coefficients and sizes. We use 513 samples on s uniformly distributed, which means

(a) (b)

(c) (d)

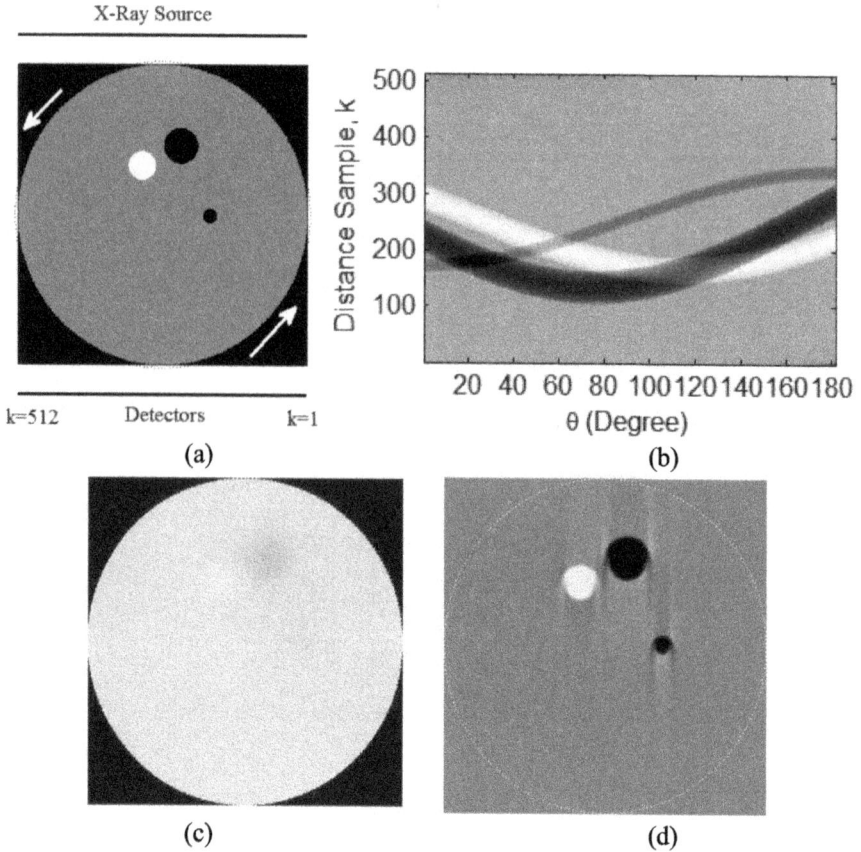

Figure 8.
A backprojection computer simulation example: (a), an intensity function $f(x,y)$ having three objects of different sizes and different absorption coefficients, position of source and detectors are at the start angle $\theta = 0$; (b), sinogram, generated by linear projection in which the distance $s = 2R$, where R is the gantry radius, is sampled into 512 samples, versus $0 \leq \theta \leq \pi$ with step 1 degree; (c), an image generated by backprojection without filtering; and (c) an image generated by filtered backprojection without filtering in which the objects are recovered.

that we can use 513 detectors uniformly distributed on the maximum width of the scanned target. Thus, each detector receives the intensity projection from the line connecting the detector to an X-ray source facing it as shown in the figure. **Figure 8(b)** shows the sinogram due to the linear projection of the intensities versus each of the rotational angle θ form 0 to 180° with a step of 1°. It is obvious that the sinogram provides information for three objects of different sizes and different absorption coefficients.

3.2.2 Fan beam projection

From **Figure 9**, we can observe that the linear projection on a detector on the arc is parameterized by the detector angle α and the rotational angle θ. Thus, the integration of the intensities of all voxels on the line $\ell(\theta, \alpha)$ is given by

$$g(\theta, \alpha) = \int_{\ell(\theta,\alpha)} f(x,y)dxdy \qquad (7)$$

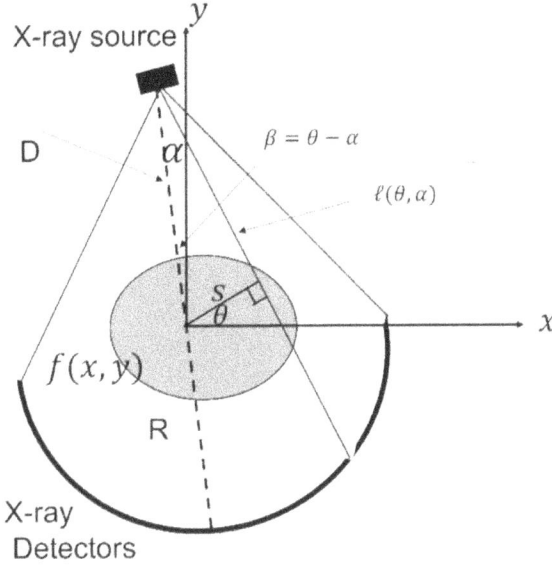

Figure 9.
An intensity function f (x, y) and the fan beam to project this intensity on an array of detectors on the arc defined by the angle $|\alpha| \leq \alpha_m$. Both the X-ray source and the detector arc rotate, simultaneously, by the angle $0 \leq \theta \leq 2\pi$, round the intensity function.

where

$$\ell(\theta, \alpha) = \{(x,y) : xcos(\theta) + ysin(\theta) = Dsin(\alpha)\} \tag{8}$$

Figure 11(a) shows a computer simulation scenario for X-Ray fan beam. The intensity function is simulated by three objects with different sizes and different absorption coefficients in a background noise. We use 257 detectors uniformly distributed on an arc of 110°, uniformly equiangular, with radius that is equal to the gantry radius, and the X-ray source position D is 1.1 of the gantry radius. **Figure 11(b)** shows the sinogram due to the projection versus the rotational angle θ from 0 to 360° with a step of 1°. It is obvious that the sinogram provides information about three objects of different sizes and different absorption coefficients.

3.3 Image reconstruction and backprojection

Backprojection aims at reconstructing an image representing an approximation of the absorption coefficient of each voxel since the true invers is not possible. In linear bean, this backprojection is given by

$$bp(x,y) = \int_0^\pi p(\theta, xcos(\theta) + ysin(\theta))d\theta \tag{9}$$

However, in fan beam, the projection is given by

$$bg(x,y) = \int_0^{2\pi} g\left(\theta, sin^{-1}\left(\frac{xcos(\theta) + ysin(\theta)}{D}\right)\right)d\theta \tag{10}$$

This implies that in both linear and fan beam projections, each (x,y)-voxel accumulates all projected values obtained from all rotational angles, which results in

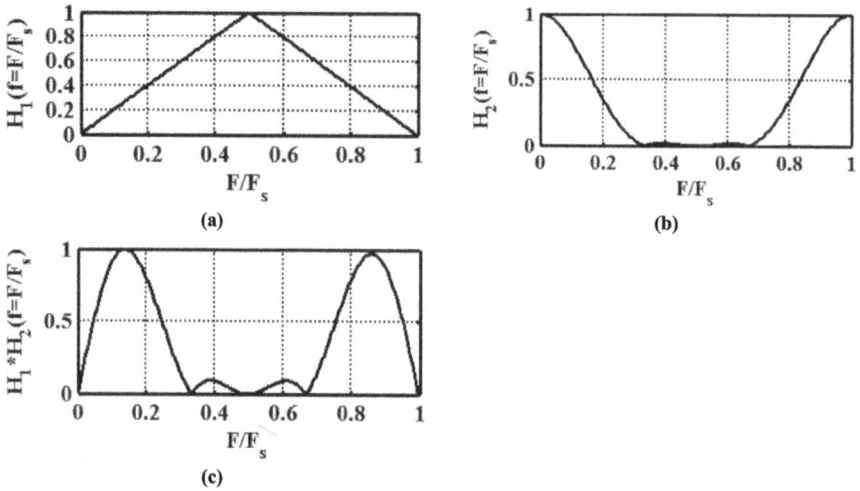

Figure 10.
Frequencies gain of three one-dimensional filters used with backprojection; (a) ramp filter; (b) low-pass filter generated by as a Hanning window; and (c), the multiplication of both filters in the frequency domain normalized to a maximum unity. The filter in (c) is sued for filtering $p(\theta, s)$ just before implementing the backprojection algorithm.

a stare-like blurring image. The voxels of true objects should have sharp intensity edges (positive or negative) compared with its neighborhoods. These sharp edges manifested themself in high frequency; this high frequency increases as the object size decreases. Thus, to remove the blurring and to enhance the resultant backprojection image, a ramp (in frequency domain) filter can be used. In such filter, the gain increases with the increase of the frequency. **Figure 10** shows in (a) the filter's amplitude versus the normalized frequency. It also shows in (b) a lowpass filter designed as a Hanning window. Finally in **Figure 10(c)**, the normalized multiplication of both filters; this resultant bandpass filter is applied to $p(\theta, s)$ just before implementing the backprojection algorithm. The algorithm employs filtering prior to backprojection, called filtered backprojection. **Figures 8(c)** and **11(c)** show the reconstructed images created by the backprojection, without filtering. It is obvious that the images are blurred, and the objects are hidden. However, **Figures 8(d)** and **11(d)** show the images obtained by the filtered backprojection. It is obvious that we get clear image in which simulated objects are manifested.

4. Medical applications

4.1 Conventional X-ray

Conventional X-ray imaging is the prompt and appropriate imaging in Emergency Department patient workup. It can prevent significant morbidity and mortality in all trauma patients. The initial and standard trauma series are X-rays of the chest, pelvis, and cervical spine. This should include systematic examination and assessment of alignment, bony structures, cartilage, and soft tissue (ABCS) [58]. In chest diseases, X-ray imaging is the first standard technique for pneumonia detection. For both viral and bacterial pneumonia. In COVID-19, conventional X-ray plays an important role as a cheap and prompt diagnostic imaging technique.

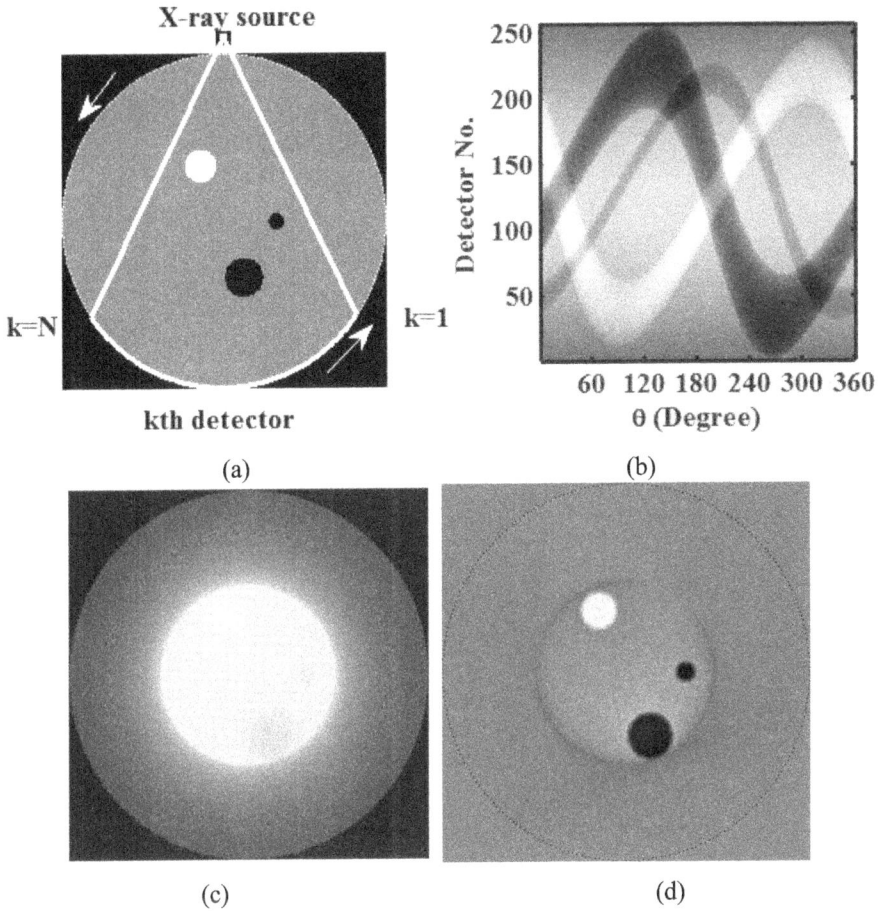

Figure 11.
A backprojection computer simulation example in fan beam- X ray and arc-shaped array of detectors: (a), an intensity function f(x,y) having three objects of different sizes and different absorption coefficients, start position at the start angle θ = 0; (b), sinogram, generated by the arc shape array detector sampled into 257 detectors (equiangular) versus the rotational angle 0 ≤ θ ≤ 2π with a step of 1 degree; (c), an image generated by backprojection without filtering; and (c) an image generated by filtered backprojection in which the objects are recovered.

Figures 12 and **13** show the use of X-ray imaging of the chest for the diagnosis of bacterial penuomnia and Covid-19.

4.2 CT scan

Low radiation load, high resolution, and fast procedure make the CT scan one of the main diagnostic tools and for different health problems. We are just interested in mentioning few CT scan application examples. CT scan could be used for detecting and screening lung carcinoma as shown in **Figure 14**. In COVID-19, CT scan has played an important role for lung instigation COVID-19-induced pneumonia. This pneumonia manifests as itself as bright spots in the image since it absorbs more X-ray energy. **Figure 15** shows in the top row non-COVID CT scan images while in the bottom one shows COVID-19 images. CT scan also is convenient imaging tool for the brain in trauma and normal clinical routine. **Figure 16** shows brain images with hemorrhage in the top row while in the bottom one shows the segmentation for detecting the hemorrhage region. Also, CT scan has been used for the investigation of spinal cord and vertebral column.

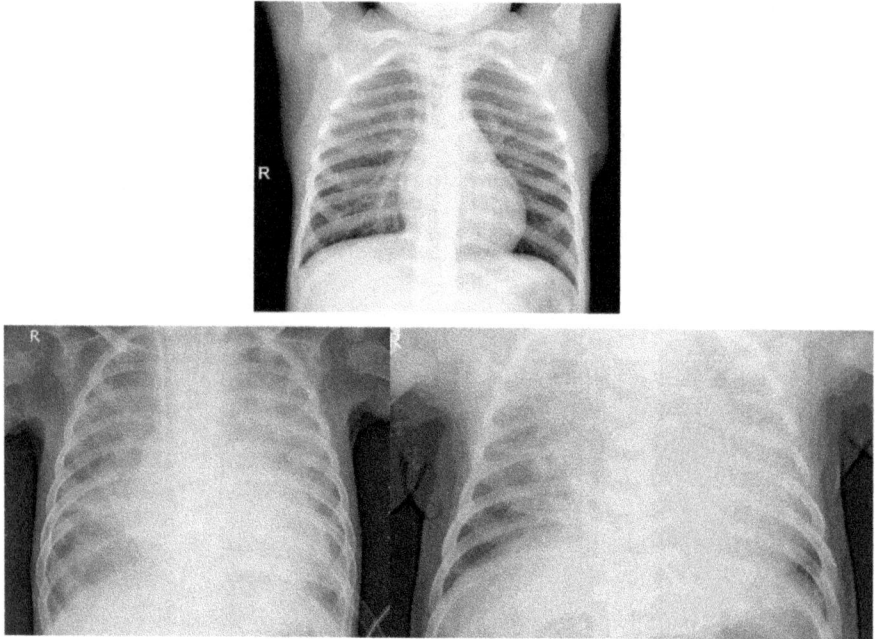

Figure 12.
Chest X-ray image. Top row, normal; bottom row, bacterial pneumonia. From Kaggel.com database: https://www.kaggle.com/tolgadincer/labeled-chest-xray-images.

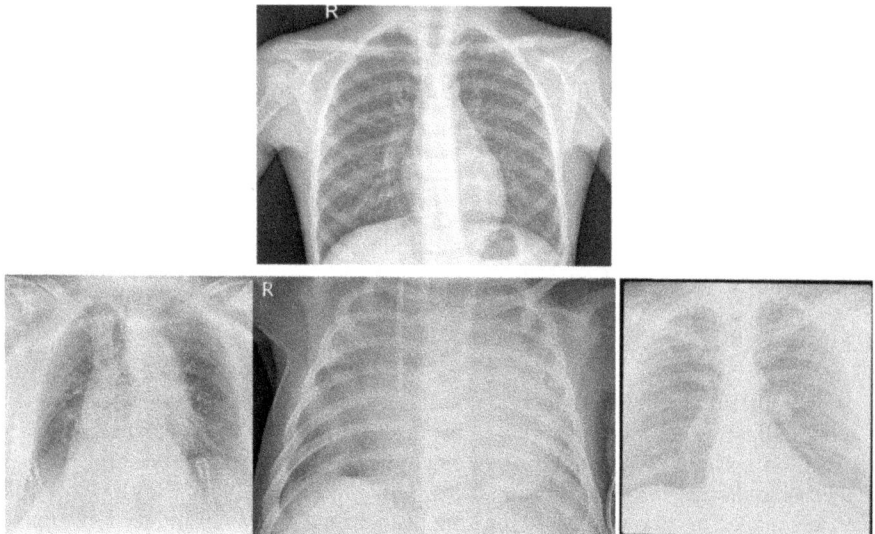

Figure 13.
Chest X-ray image. Top row, normal; bottom row, from left-to-right, COVID-19, bacterial pneumonia, and tuberculosis. From Kaggel.com database: https://www.kaggle.com/jtiptj/chest-xray-pneumoniacovid19tuberculosis

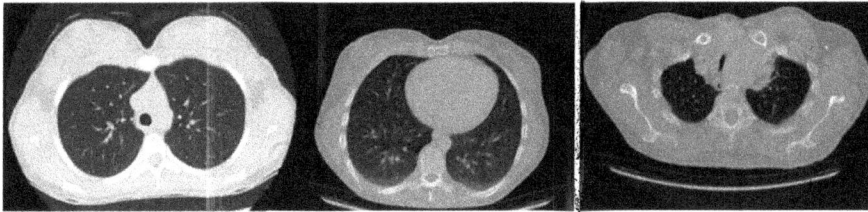

Figure 14.
Chest CT scan slices: Most left, Normal; middle, adenocarcinoma and Most right, carcinoma. From Kaggle.com: https://www.kaggle.com/mohamedhanyyy/chest-ctscan-images.

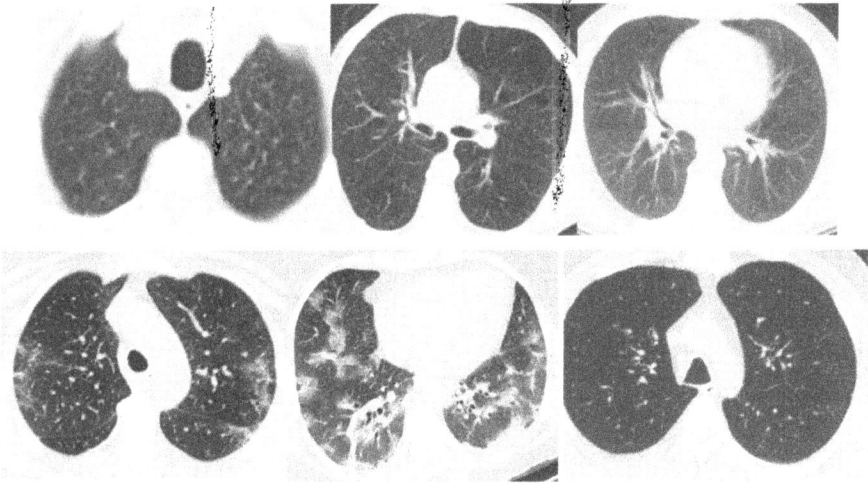

Figure 15.
Chest CT scan slices: Top row, non-COVID, bottom row, COVID. From kaggel.com: https://www.kaggle.com/plameneduardo/sarscov2-ctscan-dataset.

5. Discussion and conclusion

CT scanner has been one of the main diagnostic imaging tools in the medical field. It provides multi two-dimensional slices in the axial plane for abdomen, chest, brain, vertebral column, and spinal cord. It employs low dose of X-ray. It also takes a reasonable time to get CT scan procedure done. More work may be needed to develop CT scan technology affordable for the development countries. Appreciated research efforts are going on to mining and processing the images provided by the CT scanner to develop computer algorithms that can help in improving diagnostic accuracy. These include developing different algorithms in machine learning, image processing, statistical analysis, multi resolution analysis, fast filtered backprojection. Image processing includes noise reduction and image enhancement, features extraction, morphology analysis, image segmentation. Deep learning aims at answering a question of if disease or not disease, e.g., benign tumor or carcinoma one, COVID or non-COVID, based on the given image. In backprojection research, the objective is to develop fast and supper resolution backprojection algorithms and to employ compressive sensing for image reconstruction.

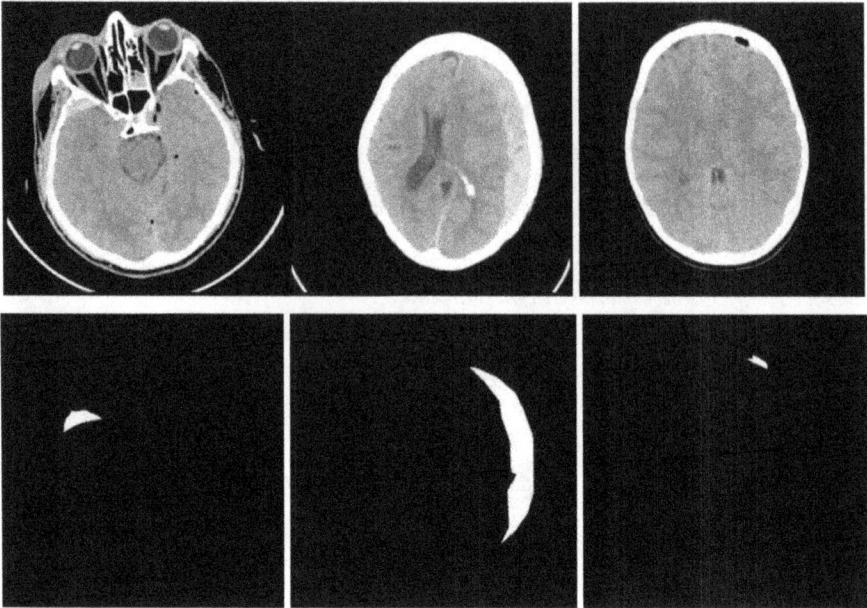

Figure 16.
Brain CT scan: Top row, brain image with intracranial Hemorrhage; bottom row, the segmentation of the image to detect the intracranial Hemorrhage region. From kaggel.com: https://www.kaggle.com/vbookshelf/computed-tomography-ct-images.e

Conflict of interest

The author declares no conflict of interest.

Author details

Reda R. Gharieb
Assiut University, Egypt

*Address all correspondence to: rrgharieb@gmail.com

IntechOpen

References

[1] Friel JJ, Lyman CE. Tutorial review: X-ray mapping in electron-beam instruments. Microscopy and Microanalysis. 2006;**12**(1):2-25

[2] Nascimento MLF. Brief history of X-ray tube patents. World Patent Information. 2014;**37**:48-53

[3] Wagner JP, Chung KC. A historical report on Robert Kienböck (1871–1953) and Kienböck's disease. The Journal of Hand Surgery. 2005;**30**(6):1117-1121

[4] Linton OW. Medical applications of x rays. Beam Line. 1995;**25**(2):25-34

[5] Pasveer B. Knowledge of shadows: The introduction of X-ray images in medicine. Sociology of Health & Illness. 1989;**11**(4):360-381

[6] Mould RF. The early history of x-ray diagnosis with emphasis on the contributions of physics 1895-1915. Physics in Medicine & Biology. 1995;**40**(11):1741

[7] Yaffe MJ, Rowlands JA. X-ray detectors for digital radiography. Physics in Medicine & Biology. 1997;**42**(1):1-39

[8] Gruner SM, Tate MW, Eikenberry EF. Charge-coupled device area X-ray detectors. Review of Scientific Instruments. 2002;**73**(8):2815-2842

[9] Bertuccio G, Caccia S, Puglisi D, Macera D. Advances in silicon carbide X-ray detectors. Nuclear Instruments and Methods in Physics Research Section A: Accelerators, Spectrometers, Detectors and Associated Equipment. 2011;**652**(1):193-196

[10] Spahn M. X-ray detectors in medical imaging. Nuclear Instruments and Methods in Physics Research Section A: Accelerators, Spectrometers, Detectors and Associated Equipment. 2013;**731**:57-63

[11] Dong Y, Pan Y, Zhang J, Xu W. Learning to read chest X-ray images from 16000+ examples using CNN. In: 2017 IEEE/ACM International Conference on Connected Health: Applications, Systems and Engineering Technologies (CHASE). Philadelphia, Pennsylvania, USA: IEEE; 2017. pp. 51-57

[12] Parveen N, Mohamed Sathik M. Detection of pneumonia in chest X-ray images. Journal of X-Ray Science and Technology. 2011;**19**(4):423-428

[13] Zhang J, Xie Y, Pang G, Liao Z, Verjans J, Li W, et al. Viral pneumonia screening on chest X-rays using confidence-aware anomaly detection. IEEE Transactions on Medical Imaging. 2021;**40**(3):879-890

[14] Ausawalaithong W, Thirach A, Marukatat S, Wilaiprasitporn T. Automatic lung cancer prediction from chest X-ray images using the deep learning approach. In: 2018 11th Biomedical Engineering International Conference (BMEICON). Thailand: IEEE; 2018. pp. 1-5

[15] Becker AS, Blüthgen C, Sekaggya-Wiltshire C, Castelnuovo B, Kambugu A, Fehr J, et al. Detection of tuberculosis patterns in digital photographs of chest X-ray images using Deep Learning: Feasibility study. The International Journal of Tuberculosis and Lung Disease. 2018;**22**(3):328-335

[16] Imran A-A-Z, Terzopoulos D. Semi-supervised multi-task learning with chest X-ray images. In: International Workshop on Machine Learning in Medical Imaging. Cham: Springer; 2019. pp. 151-159

[17] Rahman T, Khandakar A, Abdul Kadir M, Rejaul Islam K, Islam KF,

Mazhar R, et al. Reliable tuberculosis detection using chest X-ray with deep learning, segmentation and visualization. IEEE Access. 2020;**8**: 191586-191601

[18] Chandra TB, Verma K, Singh BK, Jain D, Netam SS. Automatic detection of tuberculosis related abnormalities in chest X-ray images using hierarchical feature extraction scheme. Expert Systems with Applications. 2020;**158**:113514

[19] Wu H, Xie P, Zhang H, Li D, Cheng M. Predict pneumonia with chest X-ray images based on convolutional deep neural learning networks. Journal of Intelligent & Fuzzy Systems. 2020; **39**(3):2893-2907

[20] Matsumoto T, Kodera S, Shinohara H, Ieki H. Yamaguchi T, Higashikuni Y, Kiyosue A, et al. Diagnosing heart failure from chest X-ray images using deep learning. International Heart Journal. 2020;**61**(4): 781-786

[21] Dallal AH, Agarwal C, Arbabshirani MR, Patel A, Moore G. Automatic estimation of heart boundaries and cardiothoracic ratio from chest x-ray images. In: Medical Imaging: Computer-Aided Diagnosis. Vol. 10134. USA: International Society for Optics and Photonics; 2017. p. 101340K

[22] Arndt H, Busse A, Meinel FG. Heart and lung in X-ray images: Lost art (?). Radiologe. 2020;**60**(12):1122-1130

[23] Hascoët S, Warin-Fresse K, Baruteau A-E, Hadeed K, Karsenty C, Petit J, et al. Cardiac imaging of congenital heart diseases during interventional procedures continues to evolve pros and cons of the main techniques. Archives of Cardiovascular Diseases. 2016;**109**(2):128-142

[24] Lu L, Sun RR, Liu M, Zheng Y, Zhang P. The inflammatory heart diseases: Causes, symptoms, and treatments. Cell Biochemistry and Biophysics. 2015;**72**(3):851-855

[25] Modlesky CM, Bickel CS, Slade J, Dudley GA. Assessment of skeletal muscle mass in men with spinal cord injury using dual energy X-ray absorptiometry and magnetic resonance imaging. Journal of Applied Physiology. 2004;**96**(2):561-566

[26] Parizel PM, Zijden T, Gaudino S, Spaepen M, Voormolen MHJ, Venstermans C, et al. Trauma of the spine and spinal cord: Imaging strategies. European Spine Journal. 2010;**1**(19):8-17

[27] Edwards WB, Schnitzer TJ. Bone imaging and fracture risk after spinal cord injury. Current Osteoporosis Reports. 2015;**13**(5):310-317

[28] Pearcy MJ, Whittle MW. Movements of the lumbar spine measured by three-dimensional X-ray analysis. Journal of Biomedical Engineering. 1982;**4**(2):107-112

[29] McVey G, Sandborg M, Dance DR, Carlsson GA. A study and optimization of lumbar spine X-ray imaging systems. The British Journal of Radiology. 2003; **76**(903):177-188

[30] Antani S, Rodney Long L, Thoma GR, Lee DJ. Anatomical shape representation in spine x-ray images. In: Proceedings of IASTED International Conference on Visualization, Imaging and Image Processing. 2003. pp. 510-515

[31] Jingqi JRTG. Progress of radiological research on digestive system malignancy related sarcopenia. Interventional Journal of Medical Radiology. 2020;**43**(4):457

[32] Pisano ED, Yaffe MJ. Digital mammography. Radiology. 2005; **234**(2):353-362

[33] Mazess RB, Barden HS, Bisek JP, Hanson J. Dual-energy x-ray absorptiometry for total-body and regional bone-mineral and soft-tissue composition. The American Journal of Clinical Nutrition. 1990;**51**(6):1106-1112

[34] Pietrobelli A, Formica C, Wang Z, Heymsfield SB. Dual-energy X-ray absorptiometry body composition model: Review of physical concepts. American Journal of Physiology-Endocrinology And Metabolism. 1996; **271**(6):E941-E951

[35] Hounsfield GN. Computerized transverse axial scanning (tomography): Part 1. Description of system. The British Journal of Radiology. 1973; **46**(552):1016-1022

[36] Chabat F, Yang G-Z, Hansell DM. Obstructive lung diseases: Texture classification for differentiation at CT. Radiology. 2003;**228**(3):871-877

[37] Bonelli FS, Hartman TE, Swensen SJ, Sherrick A. Accuracy of high-resolution CT in diagnosing lung diseases. AJR. American Journal of Roentgenology. 1998;**170**(6):1507-1512

[38] Johkoh T, Müller NL, Akira M, Ichikado K, Suga M, Ando M, et al. Eosinophilic lung diseases: Diagnostic accuracy of thin-section CT in 111 patients. Radiology. 2000;**216**(3): 773-780

[39] Raoof S, Raoof S, Naidich D. Imaging of unusual diffuse lung diseases. Current Opinion in Pulmonary Medicine. 2004;**10**(5):383-389

[40] Makaju S, Prasad PWC, Alsadoon A, Singh AK, Elchouemi A. Lung cancer detection using CT scan images. Procedia Computer Science. 2018;**125**:107-114

[41] Gong T, Liu R, Lim Tan C, Farzad N, Kiang Lee C, Chuan Pang B, et al. Classification of CT brain images

of head trauma. In: IAPR International Workshop on Pattern Recognition in Bioinformatics. Berlin, Heidelberg: Springer; 2007. pp. 401-408

[42] Shahangian B, Pourghassem H. Automatic brain hemorrhage segmentation and classification in CT scan images. In: 2013 8th Iranian Conference on Machine Vision and Image Processing (MVIP). IEEE; 2013. pp. 467-471

[43] Yahiaoui AFZ, Bessaid A. Segmentation of ischemic stroke area from CT brain images. In: 2016 International Symposium on Signal, Image, Video and Communications (ISIVC). IEEE; 2016. pp. 13-17

[44] Wijdicks EFM. The first CT scan of the brain: entering the neurologic information age. Neurocritical Care. 2018;**28**(3):273-275

[45] Rabinstein AA. Traumatic spinal cord injury. In: Rabinstein A, editor. Neurological Emergencies: A Practical Approach. Cham: Springer; 2020. pp. 271-280

[46] Barba CA, Taggert J, Morgan AS, Guerra J, Bernstein B, Lorenzo M, et al. A new cervical spine clearance protocol using computed tomography. Journal of Trauma and Acute Care Surgery. 2001; **51**(4):652-657

[47] Gupta PK, Krishna A, Dwivedi AN, Gupta K, Madhu B, Gouri G, et al. CT scan findings and outcomes of head injury patients: A cross sectional study. Journal of Pioneering Medical Sciences. 2011;**1**(3):78-82

[48] Kligman M, Vasili C, Roffman M. The role of computed tomography in cervical spinal injury due to diving. Archives of Orthopedic and Trauma Surgery. 2001;**121**(3):139-141

[49] Zeng GL. Image reconstruction: A tutorial. Computerized Medical Imaging and Graphics. 2001;**25**(2):97-103

[50] Hanson KM. On the optimality of the filtered backprojection algorithm. Journal of Computer Assisted Tomography. 1980;4(3):361-363

[51] Li J, Jaszczak RJ, Wang H, Coleman RE. A filtered-backprojection algorithm for fan-beam SPECT which corrects for patient motion. Physics in Medicine & Biology. 1995;**40**(2): 283-294

[52] Hiriyannaiah HP. X-ray computed tomography for medical imaging. IEEE Signal Processing Magazine. 1997;**14**(2): 42-59

[53] Wei Y, Wang G, Hsieh J. Relation between the filtered backprojection algorithm and the backprojection algorithm in CT. IEEE Signal Processing Letters. 2005;**12**(9):633-636

[54] Beister M, Kolditz D, Kalender WA. Iterative reconstruction methods in X-ray CT. Physica Medica. 2012;**28**(2): 94-108

[55] Seibert JA, Boone JM. X-ray imaging physics for nuclear medicine technologists. Part 2: X-ray interactions and image formation. Journal of Nuclear Medicine Technology. 2005;**33**(1):3-18

[56] Stanford RW, Hills TH. An advance in X-ray film processing. The British Journal of Radiology. 1956;**29**(341): 286-294

[57] Hoheisel M. Review of medical imaging with emphasis on X-ray detectors. Nuclear Instruments and Methods in Physics Research, Section A: Accelerators, Spectrometers, Detectors and Associated Equipment. 2006; **563**(1):215-224

[58] Gay DAT, Miles R. Use of imaging in trauma decision-making. BMJ Military Health. 2011;**157**(Suppl 3): S289-S292

Chapter 2

Use of Computed Tomography (CT)-Scan in the Current Coronavirus Pandemic

Ibrahima Niang, Géraud Akpo,
Khadidiatou Ndiaye Diouf and Sokhna Ba

Abstract

CT is a medical imaging technique that uses X-rays to provide three-dimensional reconstructed images of the explored anatomical region. Its sensitivity has already been demonstrated in the exploration of pulmonary lesions of traumatic, neoplastic and especially infectious origin. In this chapter we present and highlight the usefulness of CT-scan imaging for diagnosis and management of the thoracic involvement of the COVID-19 pandemic. We also present the use of CT in extra-thoracic involvement, in particular, the angio-CT of the limbs in cases of suspected arterial thrombosis of the limbs during COVID-19. Finally, we evoke the other tools such as artificial intelligence which coupled with the CT-scan allows a greater accuracy and thus are to popularize in order to reinforce the CT as a tool of first plan in the fight against future pandemics with thoracic tropism.

Keywords: CT-scan, diagnosis, coronavirus, COVID-19, ground-glass opacity, post-mortem CT, mobile CT, Artificial Intelligence

1. Introduction

Computed tomography (CT) is a diagnostic tool that uses X-rays to visualize anatomical structures of the body with a good resolution [1]. It allows the identification of abnormalities related to a pathology. It has proven itself particularly in the exploration of lung parenchyma where it has a high sensitivity in the detection of neoplastic and infectious diseases [2]. Knowing that its realization lasts only about ten seconds and that the results can be immediately available, the CT scan is a tool of choice in case of high influx of symptomatic patients and requiring triage [3]. Since the occurrence of the COVID-19 pandemic, whose main symptoms are respiratory with lung parenchymal lesions responsible for a desaturation that can be rapidly fatal, CT has taken a place of choice in the management of both suspected and confirmed cases. This is due to the fact that the reference diagnostic tool, RT-PCR on nasopharyngeal swabs, has a low sensitivity despite a good specificity [4]. Moreover, this PCR test gives results delayed by one to several days, which does not facilitate the management of patients in emergency. Thus, CT is positioned both as an emergency triage tool and as a prognostic tool to assess the extent of lung parenchymal lesions while identifying other associated lesions or other complications such as pulmonary embolism [3, 5].

2. Technique

A thoracic CT scan is performed on a patient in dorsal recumbency, with the hands placed behind the head. The patient must maintain a deep inspiration during the acquisition, which lasts about ten seconds. This acquisition must cover the whole thorax from the apex to the costo-diaphragmatic cul-de-sac. Ideally, for patients with COVID or suspected COVID, it is better to perform the examination with a dose optimization protocol (low-dose) [6]. This will reduce the cumulative irradiation dose, when we know that these patients may have to undergo several CT scans depending on their evolution.

However, the examination should be performed with injection of iodinated contrast medium, in thoracic angio-CT, when there is a clinical suspicion of pulmonary embolism [7].

3. Results

3.1 Positive diagnosis

The CT scan essentially allows the identification of the elementary lesions attributable to COVID-19, which are ground-glass opacity, crazy-paving and non-systematized condensation [8, 9].

The ground-glass opacity, which corresponds to an opacity of the lung parenchyma that does not erase the pulmonary vessels (**Figure 1A** and **B**), is the most frequent sign found in COVID-19 between 88% and 94% [9, 10].

However, ground glass opacity is a non-specific sign of COVID-19 and therefore it is above all its distribution on the lung parenchyma that is decisive for the diagnosis. In the typical form, this distribution is in bilateral sub pleural patches, predominantly in the posterior and basal regions (**Figure 1A** and **B**) [11]. However, there are less typical forms with a central, unilateral, predominantly apical or nodular distribution [10].

Crazy-paving, which corresponds to ground-glass opacity associated with thickening of the lobular septa (**Figure 2A** and **B**), is usually found in the evolution of ground-glass lesions [12].

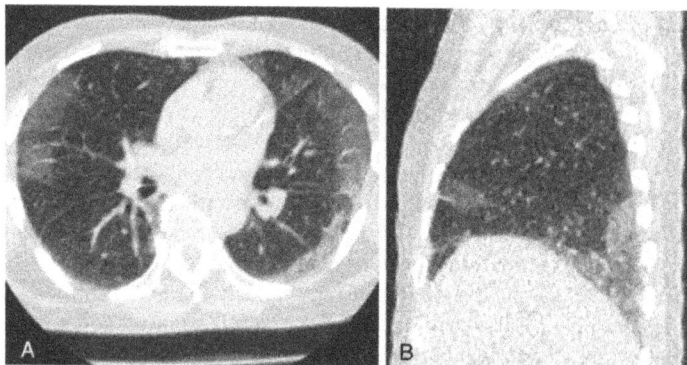

Figure 1.
Chest CT in lung window, axial section (A) and sagittal reconstruction (B) typical form of COVID-19 pulmonary lesions with bilateral areas of ground glass opacities limited to the sub pleura and predominantly at the lung bases.

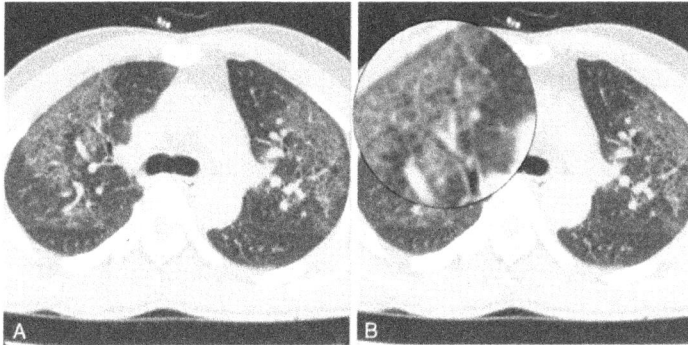

Figure 2.
Chest CT in lung window, axial sections (A and B). Thickening of the septa on a ground glass background giving the appearance of crazy-paving.

The same is true for non-systematic condensation which can occur by transformation of the initial lesions [12]. This condensation will appear as an increase in density of the lung parenchyma but unlike the ground-glass opacity, it will erase the pulmonary vessels (**Figure 3A** and **B**).

3.2 Differential diagnosis

As important as it is to know how to recognize CT signs compatible with COVID-19 infection, it is equally important to know how to differentiate it from other pathologies that require a different management and that can be life-threatening emergencies.

These differential diagnoses are first and foremost the other causes of ground-glass opacity. This is a long list covering several diffuse interstitial lung disease, acute pulmonary edema and alveolar hemorrhage among others [13]. Other causes of crazy-paving and condensation will also be a differential diagnosis, including several diffuse interstitial lung diseases, pneumonia, acute pulmonary edema, bronchioloalveolar carcinoma among others [14].

On imaging, it is important to differentiate the lesions of covid-19 with those of acute pulmonary edema and alveolar hemorrhage which are high emergencies and require specific treatment. What helps in this distinction is essentially the

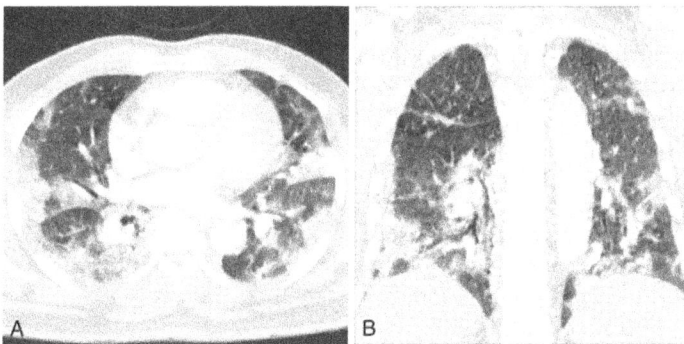

Figure 3.
Chest CT in lung window, axial section (A) and coronal reconstruction (B) bilateral patches of non-systematic sub pleural condensation, corresponding to an evolution of ground glass lesions in relation to COVID-19.

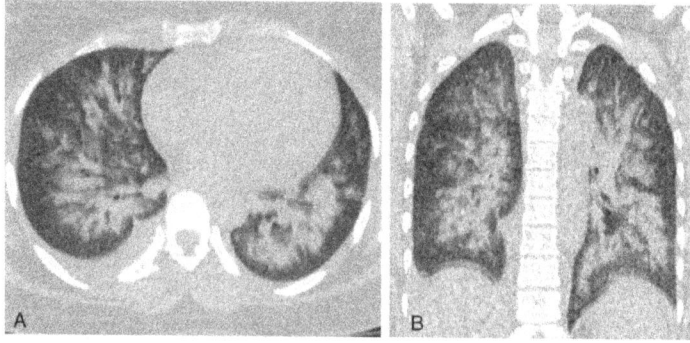

Figure 4.
Chest CT in lung window, axial section (A) and coronal reconstruction (B) bilateral areas of condensation and ground glass opacities, confluent, centrally distributed, clearly sparing the sub pleural regions. This gives the butterfly wing appearance which is in favor of pulmonary edema and rules out the suspicion of Covid-19 in the patient.

distribution of the lesions which are typically sub pleural in COVID-19 and on the contrary spares the sub pleural regions in alveolar hemorrhage and acute pulmonary edema (**Figure 4A** and **B**) [15].

However, in each case, this differential diagnosis must consider the clinical elements, the evolution and the biological data.

3.3 Severity and complications

The most important factor of severity is the degree of extent of the lesions on the lung parenchyma. A visual grading of these lung lesions has been proposed by the Society of Thoracic Imaging (STI) in five stages ranging from less than 10% involvement (minimal) to more than 75% involvement (critical) [16]. This degree of lung involvement is important to specify because it constitutes a prognostic element.

Other elements of severity are the existence of sequelae or evolving pulmonary lesions (pulmonary emphysema, sequelae of granulomatosis, active tuberculosis infection, among others).

Among the complications, the most feared and expected is pulmonary embolism [17]. The risk of embolism is high because of the significant inflammatory response during COVID-19, which makes it a highly thrombogenic pathology [18]. The search for a clinically suspected pulmonary embolism is the main indication for thoracic angio-CT in COVID-19 (**Figure 5A** and **B**) [7].

Other complications are pneumothorax and pneumomediastinum, which may occur spontaneously or as a result of mechanical ventilation [19].

Bacterial reinfection can also occur in COVID-19 pneumonia. In this case, there is a systematized condensation at a lobe or a segment, unlike the condensations related to COVID which follow the distribution of ground glass lesions, remaining sub pleural and not systematized [20].

All these elements of severity and complications influence the prognosis of the patient, which makes thoracic CT an important prognostic tool.

3.4 Evolution

The evolution of COVID-19 lung disease can be towards a regression of the lesions with possible restitution ad integrum if an adequate treatment has been

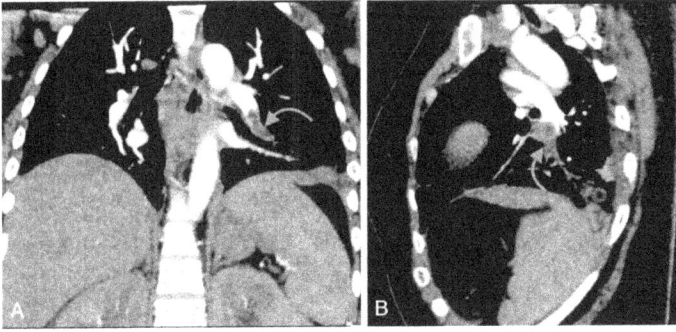

Figure 5.
Thoracic CT angiography in mediastinal window with coronal (A) and sagittal (B) reconstruction pulmonary embolism with endoluminal defect at the level of a left posterobasal segmental pulmonary artery branch (red arrows).

initiated in time. However, it should be kept in mind that regression of lesions on CT is lagging behind clinical improvement [21]. Therefore, it is important to avoid too frequent CT scans, which would be a source of unnecessary irradiation.

The evolution may also take the form of fibrosing parenchymal sequelae [21].

Furthermore, it should be borne in mind that pulmonary embolism may occur during the evolution of the disease.

4. Use of CT in extra-thoracic disease

COVID 19 is a systemic disease, although thoracic and particularly pulmonary involvement is prominent. CT can be an important tool for some of these extra thoracic conditions [22].

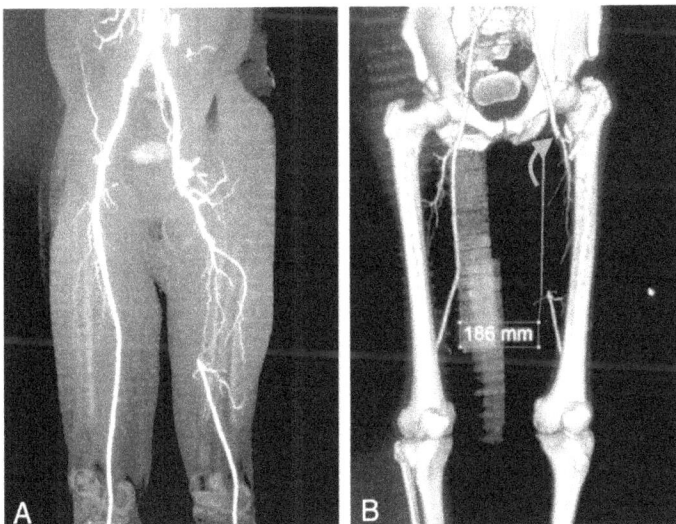

Figure 6.
Angio-CT of the lower limbs in a COVID patient with ischemia of the left lower limb. (A) Angiographic reconstruction showing the thrombosis of the superficial femoral artery from its origin (red arrow) to its lower third with revascularization by collaterals from the deep femoral artery. (B) VRT reconstruction showing the thrombosis extending over a height of 18.6 cm.

Among the extra thoracic uses of CT, we note in particular the angio-CT of the limbs in cases of suspected arterial thrombosis of the limbs during COVID-19 (**Figure 6A** and **B**).

5. Advantages and disadvantages of CT compared to other diagnostic tools

5.1 Advantages

CT has the advantage of having good spatial resolution but also availability and speed of image acquisition, which only takes about ten seconds. The reading of the images is also fast and quite easy compared to other imaging methods.

In addition, CT has good sensitivity in the detection of COVID-19 lung lesions, when compared with the reference diagnostic tool that is RT-PCR [23].

Another advantage is its contribution to the prognosis of patients by providing an overview of the lung volume affected by the lesions.

5.2 Disadvantages

The main disadvantage of CT is the irradiation, which justifies the use of dose optimization (low-dose CT) to minimize the consequences that could result from it [24].

The other disadvantage is the low specificity of lesions on CT, compared to RT-PCR. This should be considered to avoid overdiagnosis of COVID-19 on CT [23].

6. New features and perspectives

6.1 Mobile CT

The mobile CT allows to palliate the need for specialized transport of patients with or suspected of having COVID-19 for whom a CT scan is necessary. This transport may require particularly important logistics, especially for patients in intensive care [25]. For these patients, it is often easier and safer to bring a mobile device to their bedside than to move them to the imaging department, hence the importance of mobile CT in their management. And this mobile CT provides good quality images with a sensitivity that remains superior to the PCR test [25, 26].

6.2 Post mortem CT

Postmortem CT has positioned itself as an alternative to autopsy in deceased COVID-19 patients or in those suspected of having COVID-19. In these patients there is a high risk of contamination during the autopsy and this examination requires protective equipment that is not always available [27]. The thanatoradiological semiology of COVID-19 on CT is identical to that of living patients.

6.3 Artificial intelligence

Artificial intelligence is increasingly used as a means of fluidity and ease in several fields using technology, imaging and particularly CT is no exception. In the case of Covid-19, artificial intelligence associated with CT helps to make the diagnosis more accurate and also provides greater precision on the lung volume affected by the lesions [28].

7. Conclusion

This chapter has demonstrated the great usefulness of CT-scan in the fight against coronavirus pandemic, due to its rapid image acquisition, its immediate availability of results, its good spatial resolution and especially its high sensitivity in the detection of COVID-19 lesions. These assets are reinforced by mobile CT facilitating access to quality imaging in intensive care patients and the coupling with artificial intelligence tools providing greater diagnostic accuracy and assessment of lesion extent.

All of this should give CT a primary place in the response to future lung-tropic pandemics, such as the coronavirus.

Conflict of interest

The authors declare no conflict of interest.

Author details

Ibrahima Niang[1*], Géraud Akpo[1,2], Khadidiatou Ndiaye Diouf[1] and Sokhna Ba[1]

1 Radiology Department, Fann University Hospital Center, Dakar, Senegal

2 Radiology Department, Aristide Le Dantec University Hospital Center, Dakar, Senegal

*Address all correspondence to: niangibrahimaniang@gmail.com

IntechOpen

References

[1] Blum A, Walter F, Ludig T, Zhu X, Roland J. Multislice CT: Principles and new CT-scan applications. Journal of Radiology. 2000;**81**(11):1597-1614

[2] Raju S, Ghosh S, Mehta AC. Chest CT signs in pulmonary disease: A pictorial review. Chest. 2017;**151**(6):1356-1374

[3] Niang I, Diallo I, Diouf JCN, Ly M, Toure MH, Diouf KN, et al. Sorting and detection of COVID-19 by low-dose thoracic CT scan in patients consulting the radiology department of Fann hospital (Dakar-Senegal). The Pan African Medical Journal. 2020;**37**(Suppl 1):22-22

[4] Abbasi-Oshaghi E, Mirzaei F, Farahani F, Khodadadi I, Tayebinia H. Diagnosis and treatment of coronavirus disease 2019 (COVID-19): Laboratory, PCR, and chest CT imaging findings. International Journal of Surgery. 2020;**79**:143-153

[5] Albtoush OM, Al-Shdefat RB, Al-Akaileh A. Chest CT scan features from 302 patients with COVID-19 in Jordan. European Journal of Radiology Open. 2020;**7**:100295

[6] Dangis A, Gieraerts C, Bruecker YD, Janssen L, Valgaeren H, Obbels D, et al. Accuracy and reproducibility of low-dose submillisievert chest CT for the diagnosis of COVID-19. Radiology: Cardiothoracic Imaging. 2020;**2**(2):e200196

[7] Grillet F, Behr J, Calame P, Aubry S, Delabrousse E. Acute pulmonary embolism associated with COVID-19 pneumonia detected with pulmonary CT angiography. Radiology. 2020;**296**(3):E186-E188

[8] Caruso D, Zerunian M, Polici M, Pucciarelli F, Polidori T, Rucci C, et al. Chest CT features of COVID-19 in Rome, Italy. Radiology. 2020;**296**(2):E79-E85

[9] Jalaber C, Lapotre T, Morcet-Delattre T, Ribet F, Jouneau S, Lederlin M. Chest CT in COVID-19 pneumonia: A review of current knowledge. Diagnostic and Interventional Imaging. 2020;**101**(7-8):431-437

[10] Salehi S, Abedi A, Balakrishnan S, Gholamrezanezhad A. Coronavirus disease 2019 (COVID-19): A systematic review of imaging findings in 919 patients. American Journal of Roentgenology. 2020;**215**(1):87-93

[11] Goyal N, Chung M, Bernheim A, Keir G, Mei X, Huang M, et al. Computed tomography features of coronavirus disease 2019 (COVID-19): A review for radiologists. Journal of Thoracic Imaging. 2020;**35**(4):211-218

[12] Bernheim A, Mei X, Huang M, Yang Y, Fayad ZA, Zhang N, et al. Chest CT findings in coronavirus disease-19 (COVID-19): Relationship to duration of infection. Radiology. 2020;**295**(3):200463

[13] Bai HX, Hsieh B, Xiong Z, Halsey K, Choi JW, Tran TML, et al. Performance of Radiologists in Differentiating COVID-19 from Non-COVID-19 Viral Pneumonia at Chest CT. Radiology. 2020;**296**(2):E46-E54.

[14] Luo L, Luo Z, Jia Y, Zhou C, He J, Lyu J, et al. CT differential diagnosis of COVID-19 and non-COVID-19 in symptomatic suspects: A practical scoring method. BMC Pulmonary Medicine. 2020;**20**(1):129

[15] Raptis CA, Hammer MM, Short RG, Shah A, Bhalla S, Bierhals AJ, et al. Chest CT and coronavirus disease (COVID-19): A critical review of the literature to date. American Journal of Roentgenology. 2020;**215**(4):839-842

[16] COVID-19: EN DIRECT. SFR e-Bulletin; [cité 6 mars 2021]. Available

from: https://ebulletin.radiologie.fr/covid19

[17] Martínez Chamorro E, Revilla Ostolaza TY, Pérez Núñez M, Borruel Nacenta S, Cruz-Conde Rodríguez-Guerra C, Ibáñez Sanz L. Pulmonary embolisms in patients with COVID-19: A prevalence study in a tertiary hospital. Radiologia (Engl Ed). 2021;**63**(1):13-21

[18] Connors JM, Levy JH. Thromboinflammation and the hypercoagulability of COVID-19. Journal of Thrombosis and Haemostasis. 2020;**18**(7):1559-1561

[19] Shan S, Guangming L, Wei L, Xuedong Y. Spontaneous pneumomediastinum, pneumothorax and subcutaneous emphysema in COVID-19: Case report and literature review. Revista do Instituto de Medicina Tropical de São Paulo. 2020;**62**:e76

[20] Langford BJ, So M, Raybardhan S, Leung V, Westwood D, MacFadden DR, et al. Bacterial co-infection and secondary infection in patients with COVID-19: A living rapid review and meta-analysis. Clinical Microbiology and Infection. 2020;**26**(12):1622-1629

[21] Kong M, Yang H, Li X, Shen J, Xu X, Lv D. Evolution of chest CT manifestations of COVID-19: A longitudinal study. Journal of Thoracic Disease. 2020;**12**(9):4892-4907

[22] Palacios S, Schiappacasse G, Valdes R, Maldonado I, Varela C. COVID-19: Abdominal and pelvic imaging findings: A primer for radiologists. Journal of Computer Assisted Tomography. 2021;**45**(3): 352-358

[23] Ai T, Yang Z, Hou H, Zhan C, Chen C, Lv W, et al. Correlation of Chest CT and RT-PCR Testing for Coronavirus Disease 2019 (COVID-19) in China: A Report of 1014 Cases. Radiology. 2020 Aug;**296**(2):E32-E40

[24] Kang Z, Li X, Zhou S. Recommendation of low-dose CT in the detection and management of COVID-2019. European Radiology. 2020;**30**(8): 4356-4357

[25] Rho JY, Yoon KH, Jeong S, Lee JH, Park C, Kim HW. Usefulness of mobile computed tomography in patients with coronavirus disease 2019 pneumonia: A case series. Korean Journal of Radiology. 2020;**21**(8):1018-1023

[26] Liu X, Sun Z, Wang X, Chen Y, Wang L, Yu L, et al. Application of mobile helical computed tomography in combatting COVID-19. Iranian Journal of Radiology. 2021 [cité 18 sept 2021];**18**(1) Available from: https://sites.kowsarpub.com/iranjradiol/articles/106204.html#abstract

[27] De-Giorgio F, Cittadini F, Cina A, Cavarretta E, Biondi-Zoccai G, Vetrugno G, et al. Use of post-mortem chest computed tomography in Covid-19 pneumonia. Forensic Science International. 2021;**325**:110851

[28] Moezzi M, Shirbandi K, Shahvandi HK, Arjmand B, Rahim F. The diagnostic accuracy of Artificial Intelligence-Assisted CT imaging in COVID-19 disease: A systematic review and meta-analysis. Informatics in Medicine Unlocked. 2021;**24**:100591

Chapter 3

Radiation Doses and Risk Assessment during Computed Tomography of the Chest in COVID-19 Patients

Elena Ivanovna Matkevich and Ivan Vasilievich Ivanov

Abstract

Accounting for the effective dose (ED, mSv) and calculating the radiation risk during CT is necessary to predict the long-term consequences of radiation exposure on the population. We analyzed the results of 1003 CT examinations of the chest in patients with suspected COVID-19 in the city diagnostic center. The average ED and confidence intervals ($p \leq 0.05$) for patients with a single CT scan were: children (12–14 years) 2.59 ± 0.19 mSv, adolescents (15–19 years) 3.23 ± 0.17 mSv, adults (20–64 years), 3.43 ± 0.08 mSv, older persons (65 years and older) 3.28 ± 0.19 mSv. The maximum radiation risk values were $31.2 * 10^{-5}$ in women children and $29.3 * 10^{-5}$ in women adolescents, which exceeds the risk values for men in these age groups by 2.3 and 1.9 times, respectively. For the group of adult patients the risk was $11.2 * 10^{-5}$ in men and $17.4 * 10^{-5}$ in women, which is 1.6 times higher than in men. All these risk values are in the range of $10 * 10^{-5}$–$100 * 10^{-5}$, which corresponds to the level LOW. For the group of older age patients, the radiation risk was $2.6 * 10^{-5}$, which corresponds to the level of $1 * 10^{-5}$–$10 * 10^{-5}$, VERY LOW. Our materials shows in detail the technique to evaluate effective radiation doses for chest CT and calculate the radiation risk of the carcinogenic effects of this exposure.

Keywords: computed tomography, chest CT diagnostics, effective dose, radiation risks levels, the dependence of the radiation risk levels of sex and age

1. Introduction

In the coming years, due to the introduction of methods of medical diagnostics and treatment using ionizing radiation, the growth of medical exposure of the Russian population expected to continue, especially due to computed tomography (CT). Therefore, it is important to evaluate radiation dose levels and population radiation risks in the form of a possible oncological pathology among the population in the long term after exposure [1–8].

Estimating the stochastic effects on the basis of a linear non-threshold model, *P. Galle* [9] concluded that, compared to 700,000 spontaneous cancers per year, when recalculated to the French population, 7,000 deadly cancers are caused by radiation causes. Of these, 3,000 are associated with high concentrations in radon homes, 1,000- with radiation medical procedures, 10 - with radiation from the work of the nuclear industry and 1 - from increased natural radiation background. Therefore, from medical exposure, 14.3% of all radiation-related oncological pathologies arise.

Due to the widespread use of CT of the chest organs for the diagnosis of COVID-19, including during repeated examinations, this issue is of particular relevance.

The aim of the study was to assess effective radiation doses for chest CT for the diagnosis of Covid-19 and calculate the radiation risk of the effects of this exposure.

2. Material and methods

2.1 General characteristics of patients

We analyzed the results of 1003 CT examinations of the chest performed in patients with suspected COVID-19 during one week in October 2020 in the city diagnostic center. Among these patients were 6.2% children in the ages of 12–14 years old, 15.3% adolescents in the ages of 15–19 years old, 60.1% adults in the ages of 20–64 years old, and 18.4% older persons of ages 65 years and older. The average ages and confidence intervals ($p \leq 0,05$) were 13.8 ± 0.20 years old in group 1 (children), 17.1 ± 0.41 years old in group 2 (adolescents); 45.8 ± 1.47 years old in group 3 (adults) (of which 41.8% are of ages 20–45 years old and 58.2% are of ages 46–64 years old); 69.4 ± 1.79 years old in group 4 (older persons). The percentage number of male (female) persons in the groups are 51.6% (48.4%) in group 1, 52.3% (47.7%) in group 2, 46.3% (53.7%) in group 3, 47% (53%) in group 4. The proportion of patients with CT signs of pneumonia and without pathological signs amounted to a total of 54,6% and 45,4%, respectively, for each of the four age groups. The distribution of the patients into groups during CT examination is given in **Table 1**.

Groups	Age (ears)	Subgroups by patient sex	Number of patients	Proportion of patients with CT signs pneumonia, %	Proportion of patients without CT signs of pathology, %
1	Children (12–14)	1.1. Men	32	15.6	84.4
		1.2. Women	30	13.3	86.7
		1. Total	62	14.5	85.5
2	Adolescents (15–19)	2.1. Men	80	26.3	73.7
		2.2. Women	73	21.9	78.1
		2. Total	153	24.2	75.8
3	Adults (20–64)	3.1. Men	279	55.6	44.4
		3.2. Women	324	71.0	29.0
		3. Total	603	63.8	36.2
4	Older people (65 and older)	4.1. Men	87	77.0	23.0
		4.2. Women	98	51.0	49.0
		4. Total	85	63.2	36.8
Total Sample			1003	54.6	45.4

Table 1.
The distribution of patients in groups during CT examination on COVID-19.

2.2 Description of computed tomography technique, calculation of effective dose and radiation risk

CT studies of the chest were performed on a Siemens Somatom Emotion 16 scanner (16-slice) using a standard algorithm. The voltage on the tube was 130 kV with automatic modulation of the amperage; the slice thickness was 0.8 mm (pitch 1.4) or 1.5 mm (pitch 1.2). Of each patient, the values of the parameters determining the radiation load were entered into the database $CTDI_{vol}$ (mGy), DLP (mGy*cm) and ED, mSv.

The calculation of the effective dose (ED, mSv) for a single phase CT scan was performed according to the following equation.

The CTDIvol values were entered into the database from the CT scanner console. Then, the DLP was calculated by the formula:

$$DLP \, (mGy * cm) = CTDIvol \, (mGy) \, x \, irradiated \, length \, (cm) \qquad (1)$$

The procedure for registering the indicator "irradiated length (cm)" was as follows. Previously, the X-ray technician performed an X-ray (tomogram) of the chest. Then the region of interest (ROI) was installed on the CT scanner console in accordance with the Recommendations of EUR16262, 1999 [10]: Volume of investigation (routine chest) - from lung apex to the base of the lungs. The length of this area (irradiated length) was measured individually in each patient. In this area, a CT scan was subsequently performed and, accordingly, the patient was irradiated. DLP was calculated for this zone.

In our study, for the chest the "irradiated length" (Median, 25th and 75th percentile) was (cm): 31.3 (30.1–33.4) - in children, 34.7 (32.6–36.6) - in adolescents, 36.6 (34.9–38.7) - in adults, 33.3 (31.6–36.8) – for persons 65 years and older.

Then, using the DLP, the effective doses was estimated according to the formula [11]:

$$ED, mSv = K_{ED \, DLP} * DLP. \qquad (2)$$

To calculate the effective dose (ED, mSv) the chest $K_{ED \, DLP}$ conversion factor $(mSv*mGy^{-1}*cm^{-1})$ used was $K_{ED \, DLP}$ = 0.012 for both the children group (12–14 years old) and the adolescent group (15–19 years old) and $K_{ED \, DLP}$ = 0.016 for the subjects older than 19 years [12, 13].

The method of calculating the risk of radiation consequences is based on the analysis of the frequency of leukemia and other oncological diseases, hereditary disorders in subsequent generations in the population after irradiation of people during the atomic explosions in Hiroshima and Nagasaki, the Marshall Islands, after gamma irradiation of patients with cancer and after incidents and accidents at nuclear reactors. Several hundred publications with this information were summarized in ICRP Publication 103, 2007 [11], and the risks of these consequences in persons of different genders and ages were calculated depending on the radiation dose received. In our study, calculations of radiation risk are carried out according to the National Methodological Recommendations [14] as follows:

$$R = ED * r, \qquad (3)$$

where
R is the radiation risk per 100,000 population at an exposure dose of ED, mSv;
ED - effective dose, mSv;
r - risk indicator for exposure of 1 mSv (mSv^{-1}).

Age, years	Man	Woman	Age, years	Man	Woman
0–4	$5,6*10^{-5}$	$2,2*10^{-4}$	45–49	$2,9*10^{-5}$	$4,9*10^{-5}$
5–9	$5,0*10^{-5}$	$1,8*10^{-4}$	50–54	$2,6*10^{-5}$	$4,1*10^{-5}$
10–14	$4,6*10^{-5}$	$1,4*10^{-4}$	55–59	$2,1*10^{-5}$	$3,4*10^{-5}$
15–19	$4,4*10^{-5}$	$1,0*10^{-4}$	60–64	$1,7*10^{-5}$	$2,7*10^{-5}$
20–24	$4,0*10^{-5}$	$8,1*10^{-5}$	65–69	$1,3*10^{-5}$	$2,0*10^{-5}$
25–29	$3,8*10^{-5}$	$7,1*10^{-5}$	70–74	$9,5*10^{-6}$	$1,3*10^{-5}$
30–34	$3,6*10^{-5}$	$6,3*10^{-5}$	75–79	$6,4*10^{-6}$	$7,9*10^{-6}$
35–39	$3,4*10^{-5}$	$5,6*10^{-5}$	80–84	$4,3*10^{-6}$	$4,6*10^{-6}$
40–44	$3,3*10^{-5}$	$5,7*10^{-5}$	85+	$2,1*10^{-6}$	$1,3*10^{-6}$

Table 2.
Lifetime risk of death ratios, taking into account harm from reduced quality of life, calculated [14] per 1 mSv effective dose for medical diagnostic chest irradiation.

Radiation risk levels	Radiation risk	
	Values	Values per 100,000 people
NEGLIGIBLE	$<10^{-6}$ (less than 1 case per 1,000,000 people)	< 0.1
MINIMUM	10^{-6}–10^{-5} (1 to 10 cases per 1,000,000 people)	0.1–1
VERY LOW	10^{-5}–10^{-4} (1 to 10 cases per 100,000 people)	1–10
LOW	10^{-4}–10^{-3} (1 to 10 cases per 10,000 people)	10–100
MODERATE	10^{-3}–$3*10^{-3}$ (1 to 3 cases per 1,000 people)	100–300

Table 3.
The radiation risk levels (individual lifetime risk) to a patient's health associated with medical exposure during diagnostic studies or treatment procedures [14].

A risk indicator for exposure of 1 mSv used, lifetime cancer risk of radiation is $5.5 * 10^{-5}$ mSv^{-1} for the entire population regardless of age and sex. However, in this study r (risk indicator) were used, taking into account the age and sex of patients (**Table 2**) in accordance with the National Methodological Recommendations [14]. These values were calculated for the Russian population (mortality and morbidity data for 2008) using risk models and ICRP calculation methods [11, 15]. When calculating Radiation risk level, the scales listed in **Table 3** were used.

The mean and median values of effective doses in the formed groups were close, the assessment of the data according to Kolmogorov–Smirnov test for normality and Shapiro–Wilk's W test showed that the nature of their distribution is close to normal. The measured data were expressed as the average ± confidence interval (X ± CI) at p ≤ 0.05, as well as median (Me, 25th and 75th percentile). The significance of differences between the groups according to Student t-criterion, P value < 0.05 was considered for statistical significance. STATISTICA statistical software (version 10.0; Stat Soft. Inc., United States) was used for analysis.

3. Results and discussion

The average effective doses to patients with a single CT scan in the formed groups as illustrated in **Table 4** and **Figure 1A** were 2.59 ± 0.19 mSv in group 1 (children 12–14 years old), 3.23 ± 0.17 mSv in group 2 (adolescents 15–19 years

Groups	Age (years)	Subgroups by sex	ED, Me (25th; 75th percentile), mSv*	ED, X ± CI, mSv*	Radiation risk			Level
					Cases, per 100,000 people		Criteria interval	
					Calculating	Values		
1	Children (12–14)	Men	2.65 (2.45; 2.96)	2.92 ± 0.30	ED*4.6	13.4	10–100	LOW
		Women	2.17 (1.88; 2.46)	2.23 ± 0.16	ED*14.0*	31.2	10–100	LOW
		Total	2.46 (2.13; 2.70)	2.59 ± 0.19	ED*9.3*	24.1	10–100	LOW
2	Adolescents (15–19)	Men	3.38 (3.01; 3.88)	3.50 ± 0.23	ED*4.4	15.4	10–100	LOW
		Women	2.51 (2.37; 3.15)	2.93 ± 0.23	ED*10.0	29.3	10–100	LOW
		Total	3.13 (2.37; 3.60)	3.23 ± 0.17	ED*7.2	23.3	10–100	LOW
3	Adults (20–64)	Men	3.69 (3.05; 4.10)	3.61 ± 0.08	ED*3.1	11.2	10–100	LOW
		Women	3.27 (2.42; 3.77)	3.28 ± 0.13	ED*5.3	17.4	10–100	LOW
		Total	3.39 (2.72; 3.93)	$3.43 \pm 0.08^{1,2}$	ED*4.2	14.4	10–100	LOW
4	Older people (65 and older)	Men	3.15 (2.57; 3.90)	3.30 ± 0.23	ED*0.7	2.3	1–10	VERY LOW
		Women	3.26 (2.05; 4.20)	3.26 ± 0.30	ED*0.9	2.9	1–10	VERY LOW
		Total	3.21 (2.51; 3.90)	$3.28 \pm 0.19^{3,4}$	ED*0.8	2.6	1–10	VERY LOW

*Significance of differences mean values ED (X) between groups (p ≤ 0,05) [1]1 and 3, [2]2 and 3, [3]1 and 4, [4]2 and 4.

Table 4.
Effective doses and their compliance with radiation risk levels in patient groups with a single CT scan of the chest on COVID-19.

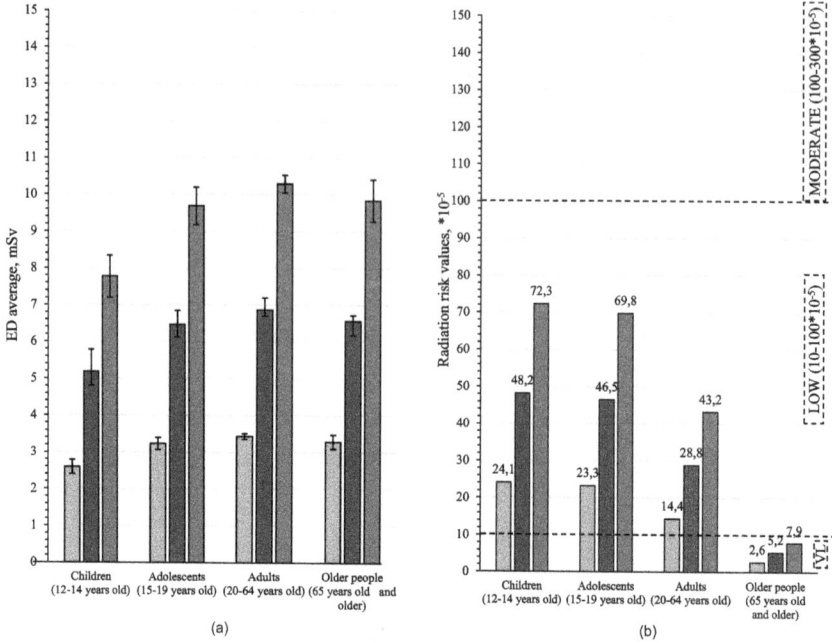

Figure 1.
Average doses, mSv (A), and radiation risk values by age groups of patients (B) with a single, double and triple computed tomography of the chest. On the ordinate axis: (A) – average effective dose and confidence intervals (p ≤ 0.05), mSv; (B) – values of radiation risk per 100,000 people; on the abscissa: age groups. Legend: number of CT scans of the patient, ▨ *– single,* ▩ *– double,* ▨ *– triple. The dashed lines show the boundaries between the levels of radiation risk (*).*

old), 3.43 ± 0.08 mSv in group 3 (adults 19–64 years old) and 3.28 ± 0.19 mSv in group 4 (older persons – 65 years and older).

These doses are comparable with the ED values shown in the report [16] on the evaluation of DRLs for adult CT in European countries and in studies of other authors [17–19]. The DRLs for CT of adult chest organs in European countries were: 4.7–6.31 mSv in Netherlands [11, 14], 5.1–5.95 mSv in Germany [16, 18], 6.8 mSv in Austria [16], 5.95–10.4 mSv in Great Britain [16, 19], 7.31 mSv in Finland [16], 8.5–10.5 in Denmark [16], as well as 7.65 mSv in Australia [20].

In our earlier study [21], with standard protocols on different CT scanners, the values of the ED were in the ranges of 2.4–6.04 mSv and 8.4–15.33 mSv, for a single-phase and multiphase with contrast CTs, respectively. The use of low-dose protocols (tube voltage from 80 to 100 kV with automatic modulation of current) made it possible to reduce the ED to 1.6 mSv, when applying the iterative reconstruction algorithm MBIR for single-phase CTs and to 4.41 mSv when applying the iterative reconstruction algorithm ASIR for multiphase CTs [22].

Based on the risk indicator value for exposure of 1 mSv with age and sex (**Table 3**) were calculations radiation risk values and radiation risk levels after chest CT radiation per 100,000 exposed persons (**Table 4**). The maximum radiation risk values for a single CT were observed (**Figure 1B**) in groups of children ($24.1*10^{-5}$) and adolescents ($23.3*10^{-5}$). As can be seen in **Figure 2B**, the radiation risk values for a single CT were $31.2*10^{-5}$ in women children (12–14 years old) and $29.3*10^{-5}$ in women adolescents (15–19 years old), which exceeds the risk values for men in these groups by 2.3 and 1.9 times, respectively. For the group of adult patients the

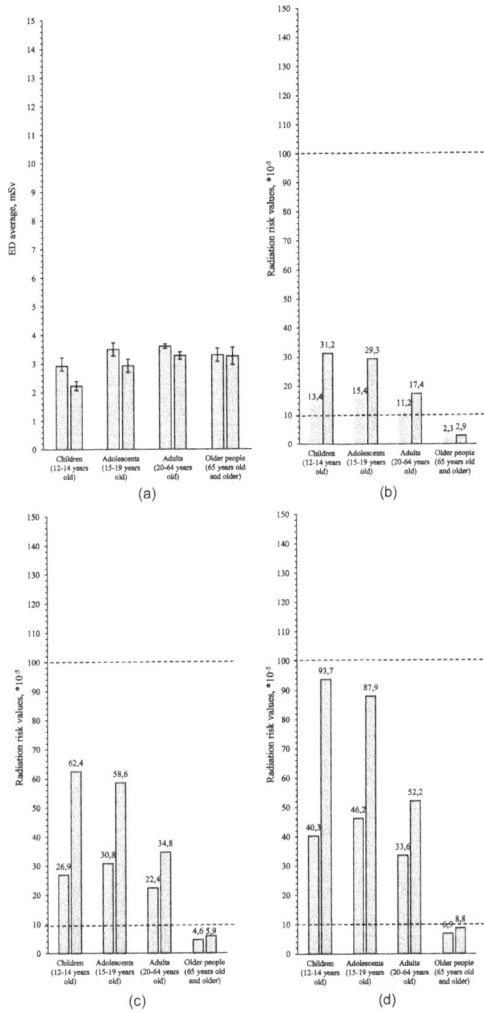

Figure 2.
Average doses for a single CT scan (A), radiation risk values for a single (B), twice repeated (C) and triple (D) CT, distribution by levels of radiation risk by age groups and depending on the sex of patients. On the ordinate axis: (A) – average effective dose and confidence intervals (p ≤ 0.05), mSv; (B–D) – values of radiation risk per 100,000 people; on the abscissa axis: age groups. Legend: – men, – women. The dashed lines show the boundaries between the levels of radiation risk (*).

average risk was $14.4*10^{-5}$, $(11.2*10^{-5})$ in men and $17.4*10^{-5}$ in women, which is 1.6 times higher than in men. Nevertheless, all these risk values are in the range of $10*10^{-5}–100*10^{-5}$, which corresponds to the level LOW. For the group of older age patients, the radiation risk was $2.6*10^{-5}$, which corresponds to the leval rang of $1*10^{-5}–10*10^{-5}$, VERY LOW.

We have compared the calculations with estimates of radiation risks in other studies.

For example, when planning the limits of exposure of astronauts [23], the risk of oncological diseases and genetic effects are rather low: $0.2*10^{-6}$ for leukemia, $0.2*10^{-6}$ for other types of malignant neoplasms, and $0.05*10^{-6}$ for genetic effects, per year per dose of additional irradiation of 1 mSv. Spontaneous incidence are

$50*10^{-6}$ for leukemia, $1000-2000*10^{-6}$ for other types of malignant neoplasms and $8000*10^{-6}$ for genetic effects per year.

In publication 103 of the ICRP [11], new views of the ICRP on the principles and approaches to ensuring radiation safety, are formulated in comparison with the previous document - Publication 60 of the ICRP [15]. Epidemiological data obtained since the publication of Publication 60 of the ICRP served as a reason for revising the values of the nominal risk factors per unit dose for radiogenic cancers and hereditary effects (**Table 5**).

As we can see, the new risk values in Publication 103 are slightly lower as those specified in Publication 60. But, at the same time, for children compared with adults, they were increased in terms of Malignant neoplasms from 1.5 to 1.68, for hereditary defects from 2.25 to 3.0, and in the total number of negative effects from 1.61 to 2.0. Our results are comparable to these guidelines.

I.A. Tsalafoutas, G.V. Koukourakis [24] emphasize that stochastic negative effects can be caused even by small doses of radiation, and give the following example of calculating the risk associated with radiation during CT. The assumption of a 5% probability of risk per 1 Sv (1,000 mSv) for the occurrence of cancer or hereditary effects means that the examination, which leads to patient exposure in ED = 10 mSv (typical for CT of the abdomen and pelvis), implies 0.05% chance of such risks. That is, for every 10,000 patients, who underwent CT with a dose of 10 mSv, five people can be expected, to develop cancer or hereditary effects as the result of radiation.

There was calculation individual of effective dose and risk of malignancy based on Monte Carlo simulations after whole body CT [25]. The Excess Relative Risk (ERR$_{MC}$), as a measurement of the exceeding risk of an exposed person compared to a non-exposed person, calculated using the solid cancer mortality in the United States as baseline (female: 17,500/100,000; male: 22,100/100,000).

There was calculation individual of Effective Dose and estimation of organ-specific additional Lifetime Attributable Risk (LAR) of cancer mortality after Whole Body Computed Tomography based on Monte Carlo simulations and report VII about Biologic Effects of Ionizing Radiation (BEIR VII). Considering the effective doses of 1.48 ± 0.15 mSv for the lungs, the LAR for mortality from lung cancer [n / 100,000] was 13.25 ± 4.24.

In our study, it was shown that with a single chest CT scan in patients with suspected COVID-19, additional (to a spontaneous level) cases of oncological pathology per 100,000 people may occur: 24.1 cases in children, 23.3 cases in adolescents, 14.4 cases in adults, 2.6 cases in older persons.

The average effective dose will increase in proportion to the increase in the number of CTs performed on the patient from 2.6–3.4 mSv with a single CT scan to the calculated values of 7.8–10.3 mSv with three times CTs. This will lead to a threefold increase in radiation risks to levels per 100,000 people may occur

Irradiated population	Malignant neoplasms		Hereditary effects		Total	
	Publ. 103	Publ. 60	Publ. 103	Publ. 60	Publ. 103	Publ. 60
Whole population	5.5	6.0	0.2	1.3	6.0	7.3
Adults	4.1	4.8	0.1	0.8	4.0	5.6
Children	6.9	7.2	0.3	1.8	8.0	9.0
K$_{Adults/\ Children}$	1.68	1.5	3.0	2.25	2.0	1.61

Table 5.
Comparison of the risk of negative effects of exposure from a dose of 1 mSv, number of cases per 10^5 people (ICRP Publication 103, 2007 [11]; ICRP Publication 60, 1991 [15]).

(**Figure 1B**): 72.3 cases in children, 69.8 cases in adolescents, 43.2 cases in adults, 7.9 cases in older persons. Due to the increased post-radiation risks in children; ccurrently, both the European and the American Society of Pediatric Radiology do not recommend the use of CT to diagnose COVID-19 pneumonia in children. CT is indicated only for severe, where concurrent pathology need to be excluded.

In men, the average radiation doses in the four age groups were slightly higher than in women (**Figure 2A**). However, with an increase in the number of CT scans from one (**Figure 2B**) to two (**Figure 2C**) and up to three (**Figure 2D**) in females, the increase in the calculated radiation risk compared to men is more significant, especially in women children (in 2.3 times) and among women adolescent (in 1.9 times). The radiation risk in men and women in all subgroups by age up to 65 years remains at the LOW level ($10*10^{-5}$–$100*10^{-5}$), and in the older subgroup at the WERY LOW level ($1*10^{-5}$–$10*10^{-5}$). However, with a three-fold CT scan in groups of children and adolescents, the radiation risk in women approaches the border of the MODERATE level ($100*10^{-5}$–$300*10^{-5}$), and in the old group to the border of the LOW level ($10*10^{-5}$–$100*10^{-5}$).

By evaluating the lung irradiation with the doses used in the ongoing clinical trials to treat COVID -19 patients, our data shows that a radiation dose 0.5 Gy provides an acceptable Risk Identification Checklist (RIC) estimate (LAR 1%), irrespective of sex and age at exposure [26]. However, a promising direction is the use of modern CT scanners, which allow the use of low-dose algorithms for CT diagnostics [27], while significantly reducing the radiation exposure to patients.

4. Conclusions

Because the study established effective radiation doses for chest CTs of patients with the diagnosis of COVID-19, the radiation risks for a single, double and triple chest CTs in different age and sex of patients were calculated. It has been found, that the radiation risk due to a single, double and triple chest CTs for patients under 65 years old is LOW, and for 65 years old and older patents is VERY LOW. Taking into account the radiation risk during CT is necessary to reduce the long-term consequences of radiation exposure on the population.

Financing

The study was performed without external funding.

Conflict of interest

The authors declare no conflict of interest.

Conformity with the principles of ethics

The study was approved by the local ethics committee.

Abbreviations

ASIR	Adaptive Statistical Iterative Reconstruction
CT	Computed tomography

CTDI$_{vol}$	Computed tomography dose index
DLP	Dose length product
DRLs	Diagnostic reference levels
ED	Effective doses
ICRP	International Commission on Radiological Protection
LAR	Lifetime Attributable Risk
MBIR	Model-Based Iterative Reconstruction

Author details

Elena Ivanovna Matkevich and Ivan Vasilievich Ivanov[*]
Department of Occupational Health, I.M. Sechenov First Moscow State Medical University of the Ministry of Health of the Russian Federation (Sechenov University), Moscow, Russian Federation

[*]Address all correspondence to: ivanov-iv@yandex.ru

IntechOpen

References

[1] Demin VF, Biryukov AP, Sedankin MK, Solov'ev VY. Specific risk of radiogenic cancer for professionals. Medical radiology and radiation safety. 2020;65(2):17–20. (In Russ.). DOI:10.12737/1024-6177-2020-65-2-17-20.

[2] Linet MS, Slovis ThL, Miller DL, Kleinerman R, Lee Ch, Rajaraman P, et al. Cancer risks associated with external radiation from diagnostic imaging procedures. 2012; CA: Cancer J Clin. 62(2):75–100. DOI:10.3322/caac.21132.

[3] Smith-Bindman R, Lipson J, Marcus R, Kim K-P, Mahesh M, Gould R, et al. Radiation dose associated with common computed tomography examinations and the associated lifetime attributable risk of cancer. 2009; Arch Intern Med. 169(22):2078–86. DOI: 10.1001/archinternmed.2009.427.

[4] Mathews J.D., Forsythe A.V., Brady Z., Butler M.W., Goergen S.K., Byrnes G.B., et al. Cancer risk in 680000 people exposed to computed tomography scans in childhood or adolescence: data linkage study of 11 million Australians. BMJ. 2013;346: f2360–f2378. DOI:10.1136/bmj.f2360.

[5] Brenner DJ, Elliston C, Hall E, Berdon W. Estimated risks of radiationinduced fatal cancer from pediatric CT. Am J Roentgenol. 2001; 176(2):289–296. DOI:10.2214/ajr.176.2.1760289.

[6] Hall EJ, Brenner DJ. Cancer risks from diagnostic radiology. Br J Radiol. 2008;81(965):362–378, DOI:10.1259/bjr/01948454.

[7] Hendee WR, O'Connor MK, Radiation risks of medical imaging: separating fact from fantasy. Radiology. 2012;264(2)312–321. DOI:10.1148/radiol.12112678.

[8] Cardis E, Howe G, Ron E, Bebeshko V, Bogdanova T, Bouville A, et al. Cancer consequences of the Chernobyl accident: 20 years on. J Radiol Prot. 2006:26(2)127–140. DOI: 10.1088/0952-4746/26/2/001. PMID: 16738412.

[9] Galle P. The Sievert: an Enigmatic Unit. Cell. Mol. Biol. (Noisy-le-grand). 2001:47(3)565–7. PMID: 11441965.

[10] EUR16262, 1999. European guidelines on quality criteria in Computed Tomography. Brussels, Belgium: European Commission, Report EUR 16262. 1999. Available via: https://op.europa.eu/da/publication-detail/-/publication/d229c9e1-a967-49de-b169-59ee68605f1a. (Accessed 17 August 2021).

[11] ICRP, 2007. The 2007 Recommendations of the International Commission on Radiological Protection. ICRP Publication 103. Ann. ICRP 2007; 37(2–4):1-332. https://www.icrp.org/publication.asp?id=ICRP%20Publication%20103 (Accessed 17 August 2021).

[12] Methodical guidelines MUK 2.6.7.3652-20. 2.6.7. Ionizing radiation, health status of workers and population. Control methods in CT diagnostics to optimize radiation protection. Moscow, 2020. https://www.rospotrebnadzor.ru/documents/details.php?ELEMENT_ID=15989&sphrase_id=2970544 (Accessed 17 August 2021). (In Russ.).

[13] Methodical guidelines MU 2.6.1.2944-11. Ionizing radiation, radiation safety. Monitoring of the effective doses of patient due to medical x-ray examinations. Moscow, 2011. (Edition of MU 2.6.1.3584-19, 10.30.2019) https://www.rospotrebnadzor.ru/documents/details.php?ELEMENT_ID=15996&sphrase_id=2970477 (Accessed 17 August 2021). (In Russ.).

[14] Assessment of radiation risk in patients during X-ray and radiological studies: Methodical recommendations MR 2.6.1.0215-20. Moscow, 2020. https://www.rospotrebnadzor.ru/documents/details.php?ELEMENT_ID=15991&sphrase_id=2970473 (Accessed 17 August 2021). (In Russ.).

[15] ICRP, 1991. 1990 Recommendations of the International Commission on Radiological Protection. ICRP Publication 60. Ann. ICRP 21; 1991; 1–3: 1-211. http://www.icrp.org/publication.asp?id=ICRP%20Publication%2060 (Accessed 17 August 2021).

[16] Damilakis J., Frija G., Hierath M., Jaschke W., Mayerhofer-Sebera U., Paulo G, et al. European Study on Clinical Diagnostic Reference Levels for X-ray Medical Imaging. Deliverable 2.1: Report and review on existing clinical DRLs. March 2018. http://www.eurosafeimaging.org/wp/wp-content/uploads/2017/09/D2.1_Report-and-review-on-existing-clinical-DRLs_final_published-on-website.pdf. (Accessed 17 August 2021).

[17] Molen AJ, Schilham A, Stoop P, Prokop M, Geleijns J. A national survey on radiation dose in CT in The Netherlands. Insights Imaging. 2013; 4 (3):383–390. DOI: 10.1007/s13244-013-0253-9.

[18] Bekanntmachung der aktualisierten diagnostischen Referenzwerte. Bekanntmachung der aktualisierten diagnostischen Referenzwerte für diagnostische und interventionelle Röntgenuntersuchungen. Tabelle 7: Diagnostische Referenzwerte für Computertomographie (CT)-Untersuchungen am Erwachsenen 22 Juni 2016. https://www.bfs.de/DE/themen/ion/anwendung-medizin/diagnostik/referenzwerte/referenzwerte_node.html. (Accessed 01 August 2021).

[19] Shrimpton PC, Hillier MC, Lewis MA, Dunn M. National survey of doses from CT in the UK: 2003. Br. J. Radiol. 2006; 79(948):968–980. DOI: 10.1259/bjr/93277434.

[20] Hayton A., Wallace A., Marks P., Edmonds K., Tingey D & Johnston P. Australian diagnostic reference levels for multi detector computed tomography. Australas. Phys. Eng. Sci. Med. 2013;36(1):19–26. DOI:10.1007/s13246-013-0180-6.

[21] Matkevich EI, Sinitsyn VE, Bashkov AN, Comparison of Radiation Dose of Patients During Single-phase and Multiphase Computed Tomography in the Multidisciplinary Treatment Clinic. Medical Radiology and Radiation Safety. 2016;61(6)50–6. http://medradiol.fmbafmbc.ru/vypuski?id=231. (Accessed 17 August 2021). (In Russ.).

[22] Matkevich EI, Sinitsyn VE, Zelikman MI, Kruchinin SA, Ivanov IV. Main directions of reducing patient irradiation doses in computed tomography. Russian Electronic Journal of Radiology (REJR). 2018;8(3):60–73. DOI: 10.21569/2222-7415-2018-8-3-60-73. (In Russ.).

[23] Grigoriev YuG. Long-term effects of radiation damage. In: Radiation safety of space flights. Radiobiological aspects. Moscow, Atomizdat, 1975, P. 40–4. (In Russ.).

[24] Tsalafoutas IA, Koukourakis GV. Patient dose considerations in computed tomography examinations. World J. Radiol. 2010;2(7):262–268, DOI: 10.4329/wjr.v2.i7.262.

[25] Kopp M, Loewe T, Wuest W, Brand M, Wetzl M., Nitsch W, et al. Individual calculation of effective dose and risk of malignancy based on Monte Carlo simulations after whole body Computed tomography. Scientific Reports. 2020;10,9475. DOI: 10.1038/s41598-020-66366-2.

[26] Arruda GA, Weber RRS, Bruno AC&Pavoni JF. The risk of induced

cancer and ischemic heart disease
following low dose lung irradiation for
COVID-19: estimation based on a virtual
case. International Journal of Radiation
Biology. 2021;97(2):120–125. DOI:
10.1080/09553002.2021.1846818.

[27] Matkevich EI, Sinitsyn VE,
Ivanov IV. Optimization of radiation
exposure in computed tomography.
Moscow-Voronezh: Elist, 2018.
(In Russ.).

Chapter 4

PET-CT Imaging and Applications

Sikandar Shaikh

Abstract

PET-CT is an important imaging modality which is well established in the recent years. The role of the molecular imaging in the evaluation of the various pathologies has been increased due to the various technological advances, radiotracer advances and also in the research. This chapter is emphasised to give the broader and better overview of the PET-CT imaging which will be used for various applications in broader fields. These advanced imaging techniques will form the basis of the different clinical applications of the PET-CT. Thus, there will have more precise applications in various pathologies which will increase the sensitivity and specificity of the different disease processes. The understanding of the basic techniques is important before being used in various pathologies. The techniques can be routine or special like the puff cheek technique for the better evaluation of the oral malignancies. The newer concept of the dual time point imaging which is being used to differentiate between the various infective and inflammatory lesions from the malignant pathologies. This chapter emphasises the use of the various techniques for various focussed clinical applications.

Keywords: molecular imaging, PET, CT, radiotracer, fluorodeoxyglucose FDG, photo multiplier tube PMT, uptake

1. Introduction

The Society of Nuclear Medicine and Molecular Imaging has defined molecular imaging as "the visualisation, characterisation, and measurement of biological processes at the molecular and cellular levels in humans and other living systems. This PET-CT imaging is based on two important software aspects two-dimensional (2D) or three-dimensional (3D) imaging techniques which are useful for the evaluation of various pathologies. The basis here is that the newer PET-CT machines are having more 3D software which is capable of better resolution. The use of the positron emission tomography (PET) by using the 18F-fluoro-2-deoxy-D-glucose as the radiotracer forms the basis of the modern imaging newer concepts leading to the personalised medicine.

The development of the PET instrumentation is based on the early development in the radioisotope manufacture in the radiochemistry. This was in the 1970s, where the Ter-Pogossian and colleagues [1] has mentioned the different compounds in the article in Scientific American which are 15O, 13N, 11C, or 18F. Along with this the FDG was also one of the compounds which was developed in first half of the 1970s at the Hospital of the University of Pennsylvania (PENN) by the Martin Reivich, David Kuhl, and Abass Alavi and also at the Brookhaven National Laboratory (BNL) [2]. The first PET center in PENN was established in August 1976, and FDG was used as the radiotracer. This was the first of the machine with the low-energy

Positron Emission Tomography (PET) Scanner

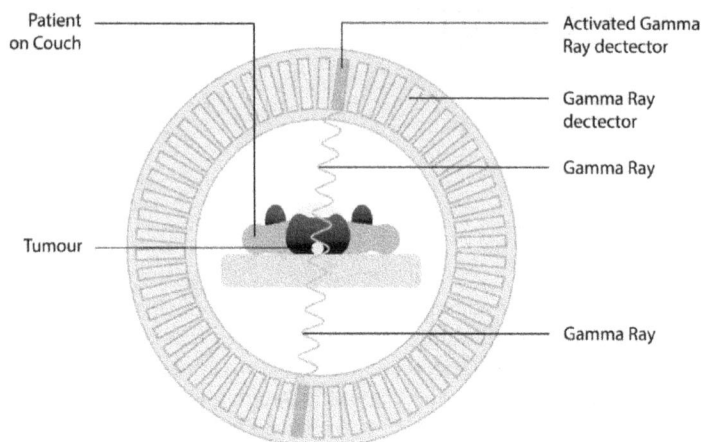

Figure 1.
The PET gantry showing the patient surrounding the gantry with scintillators surrounding the patient. The activated gamma camera with gamma rays passing through this ray.

gamma photons and this was later modified into the high-energy collimators which are capable of the positron emission photons. And thus, the first whole-body image was acquired with a dual-head rectilinear scanner comprising of the high-energy collimators. This PET III scanner was shifted to the University of the Pennsylvania (**Figure 1**) [3–6].

2. Positron emission tomography technology

2.1 PET annihilation

The first use of the PET in the imaging was done by the use of the various short-lived positron-emitting isotopes like 11C, 13N, 15O, and 18F which are being produced as generator-produced gallium 68 (68Ga) and rubidium 82 (82Rb). The production of these isotopes is done by the use of the proton irradiation of the various natural or enriched targets, and all these will be having the various production equation, half-lives, and also the various properties of the positron-emitting radionuclides. The positron emission is the process which is also the beta plus decay (b1 decay), also known as the isobaric decay process in which the proton will be converted into a neutron by releasing a positron and a neutrino. And this decay process is made up of the proton-rich radionuclides. The use of the positron decay will be resulting in the formation of the element which will be having the atomic number which will be less by one unit. This process is known as the nuclear transmutation where there will be the conversion of one isotope or the element into the another. Thus, the isobaric decay process will be representing the mass number of the daughter nuclei which will be the same, but the atomic number will be changing.

Here the process in which the proton-rich radionuclides will be converting into the stable nuclei by the isobaric decaying of the element resulting into the positron emission or electron capture. There will be the proton rich nuclide which are capable of the absorption of the inner shell electron where there will be the conversion of the proton into the neutron. This is the process where the insufficient energy will be having difference with the element as well as the prospective daughter. The minimum energy difference here is if less than 1.022 MeV, the positron emission is not possible. The electron capture here will be in the usual decay mode. The positron emission is common in the lower atomic-weight nuclei made up of the 11C, 13N, 15O, and 18F, and the electron capture is seen in iodine 123.

The positron is capable of the moving into the very short distance and is seen as Positron energy 1 neutrino energy with the 5-transition energy of the 1.022 MeV. During this process the electron clouds due to the various surrounding materials will be retarding the energy, this along with the electron system will be forming the positronium which is the unstable system made up of the electron and a positron. These components will annihilate each other within the fraction of the second like 125 picoseconds to produce the various annihilation photons having energy equivalent of 511 keV. This is the energy which will be equivalent to the combined mass of the electron and a positron, and this is emitted in opposite directions most of the times at 180 degrees to each other (**Figure 2**).

These annihilation photons which are being emitted at 180 are being detected by PET detectors by the principle of electronic collimation. The arrival of the annihilation photons here is based on the very small timing of the window which is usually the 3–15 nanoseconds. This process will be resulting into the process of the coincidence detection in PET. These detection at 180 is resulting in the formation of the line of the response which is the straight line drawn between the 2 detectors, and this process is the line of response (LOR) or coincidence line. The common availability of the various detectors having the faster timing decay, along with the high light output, and also the higher stopping power. The use of the PET scanners having the time-of-flight (TOF) capability thus it will be resulting the principle of which relies on measuring the arrival time difference of the 2 annihilation photons. The pinpoint emission point is also seen along the LOR. The ultimate use of the TOF will result in the better contrast PET images having the better sensitivity [7]. The TOF position will be resulting the along the LOR is clearly defined and resulting into the various coincidence time resolution.

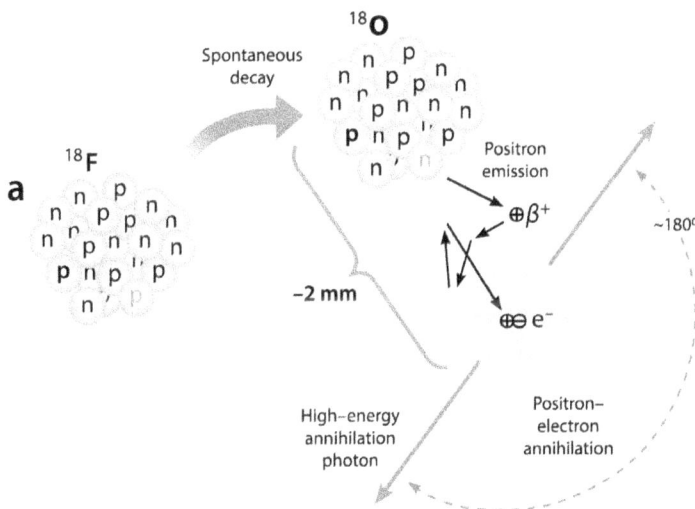

Figure 2.
This showing the principle of the positron emission where the beta decay causing the positron electron annihilation at 180 degree.

2.2 PET-scan

These scanners are made up of the various many small detectors which are usually placed in adjacent rings around the patient. The clinical state-of-the-art PET system was having a ring diameter of 60–90 cm with the extent of 10–25 cm and made up to 25,000 detectors. The single PET detector is made up of the very high-density scintillator crystal (eg, BGO, lutetium yttrium orthosilicate [LSO], or lutetium yttrium orthosilicate [LYSO]) which are capable of converting the photons striking on the detector into light. The scintillator is usually optically coupled to a device, of which the photo multiplier tube (PMT) is the commonly seen where the light will be converted into an amplified electric signal (**Figure 3**). These signals arising from the single detector will be added the coincidence circuit and this will be added as the PET event identified by the detection time. These various photons which are being detected within these various coincidence windows are documented as the coincidence events which will be attached to the LOR having the various 2 detectors, and all these events will be rejected.

Majority of these PET systems will be acquiring the data over a given time frame and these events will be tagged with the LOR position and also at the time point of detection.

The tomographic single slice is being reconstructed independently by only accepting LOR within the given slice. These independent reconstructions are being obtained by using the various lead or tungsten collimating rings in between crystal rings and these inter-ring coincidences can be prevented. This process of the imaging is called 2D PET. The higher sensitivity of the inter-ring coincidences will be resulting into the 3D PET. Usually the 2D PET is preferred over 3D PET as it is easier to have simple data for handling and various image reconstruction algorithms. But due to the various technological development having the better iterative reconstruction algorithms the sensitivity from 3D PET is now more preferred in the various clinical PET systems. The various 511-keV photons from the various annihilation events are being detected in the PET system which are within the coincidence window, and these are being referred as the random coincidences. These random

PET Scanner

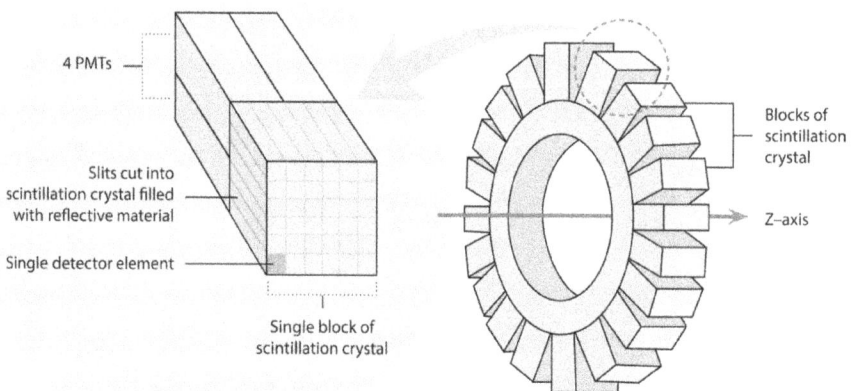

Figure 3.
Image showing the blocks of the scintillating crystals which will be showing the multiple bocks of the PMTs, and each block of the scintillation crystal are made up of the 4 PMTs.

coincidences in LOR will define the width of the coincidence window and also the various event rates in the detectors which will be defining the LOR. These will result in the various random coincidences being modelled by the various coincidence effects.

2.3 Developments in PET instrumentation

Due to the various quantitation of the smaller lesions due to the increased image contrast and along the various partial volume effects. These limitations of the PET reconstructed spatial resolution of close to the 5 mm will be resulting in various partial volume effects. This spatial resolution is based on the various size of the detector crystals, where the spatial resolution can be improved with the use of the smaller crystals. In the older versions of the conventional PET designs, the light output from a particular crystal is being shared by the use of the several PMTs. These improvements in spatial resolution will have the direct electronic readout of the light emitted by a given crystal. These features will be seen in the PET photon-counting detector designs [8] and also in PET detectors where the silicon photomultiplier detectors are being developed and also used for PET/MR imaging [9].

The modern PET systems are made up of the TOF capabilities which will be having the biggest advantage of better image contrast, resolution with the improved noise which will be further reduced by the better localization of the annihilation position. The TOF resolution is directly related to the with the growth in the technology the signal-to-noise ratio in the new detector designs will be having better TOF resolution. The improvements in signal-to-noise ratios will be reducing the less activity as well as the scan time in each patient. There is the potential reduction in the patient dose or PET scan time which will be increasing the PET scanner sensitivity, and this is based on the advancements and improvements of the various PET detector.

2.4 PET radionuclides

FDG production 18F is produced in a cyclotron by the process of the nuclear reaction between oxygen 18 (18O)-enriched water which is being bombarded with protons by the releasing of the neutron. In the 68Ga, the germanium 68 which will be bound to the generator will result into another daughter isotope.

The half-life of 110 minutes is the ideal one for the clinical use and this will be used for the synthesis which can be used for hours. The very low positron energy (640 keV) will be resulting in the very short tissue range (2.3 mm) causing the higher resolution and low radiation dose. The 18F synthesis for the higher radioactive material will be having the advantages over the short-lived radioisotopes and also for the plasma analysis which will be needed for the quantification as well as for the evaluation.

2.5 The FDG concept

The basis of the tumour metabolism is that they consume more energy in the form of the glucose as this is the most commonly used metabolite, this happens by the process of the increased glycolysis which is also known as Warburg effect. This is the principle which is being used in the PET when FDG is used as a radiotracer. The FDG is a radiolabelled glucose analogue in which the 20-hydroxyl group is being substituted by 18F.

Many factors will be having an impact on the glycolysis of the tumour cells like the histologic type, the tumour grading, the tumour cell proliferation and most important is the tumour vasculature all these factors are important for the delivery of glucose and oxygen to the tissues [10]. The less amount of the oxygenation will result in the tumour hypoxia, and this is being explained on the basis of the tumours with the lower partial pressure of oxygen in comparison to the normal tissues. The tumour hypoxia will also be based on the principle of the solid tumours. The detection of the hypoxic regions means more malignant potential with bad prognosis and resistance to the therapy [11].

The increased glucose and also the hyperinsulinism will be resulting in the less amount of the FDG uptake in the tumours based on the uptake of FDG and glucose which will be competing with each other. This is the reason that the at least 4–6 hours fasting is needed before the FDG injection which will reduce insulin levels and will be facilitating the better background ratio. For the evaluation of the various pathologies the blood glucose levels have to be within normal range, 150–200 mg/dL. If the sugar levels are more than these values, then the PET-CT should be rescheduled unless and until it is stabilised to normal levels. The reason for this is that the insulin-induced hypoglycaemia will show the less tumour uptake and also facilitates the normal physiological uptake in the muscles and fat, causing the significant reduction of the tumour-to background ratio.

The normal uptake which appears more prominent in the brain and the heart due to increased glycolysis. In the cerebral parenchyma it will be more uniform in the cortex and basal ganglia, and corresponding lesser uptake in white matter and in the cerebrospinal fluid. The myocardial uptake is significantly variable can be very high, low, or absent also. This pattern is seen in the left ventricle; however, the right ventricle and atria uptake are not very high (**Figure 4**). The prolonged fasting of the 18 hours or more and a the low-carbohydrate-high-fat diet will result

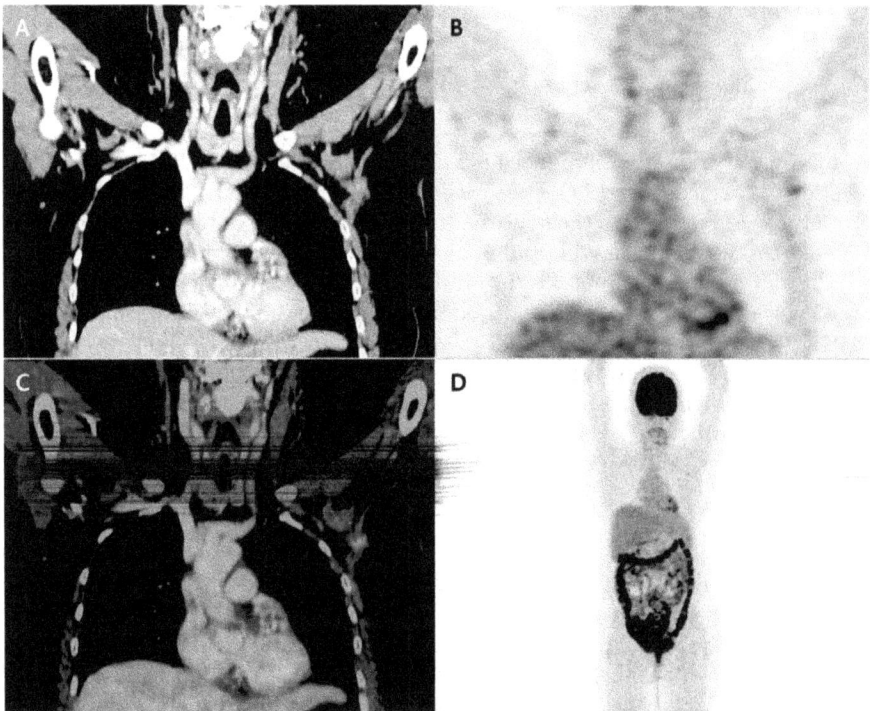

Figure 4.
This PET-CT images (a–c) showing the normal mild physiological uptake, image (d) showing the physiological uptake in the bowel loops in the whole body scan.

in the change of the metabolism like glucose to free fatty acids, this will result into the varied uptake due to the temporal and geographic diversities of the decreased glycolytic activity. The normal physiologic uptake in the various organs like the liver, spleen, and bone marrow are usually homogenous and low; on contrary the bone marrow will be showing significant uptake in following conditions like systemic inflammation, prolonged bleeding, or associated therapeutic interventions with chemotherapy or bone marrow stimulants. With this pattern of the uptake the different types of the skeletal metastases or associated malignant bone marrow infiltration; and this will result in the skeletal metastases.

Another important aspect of is that the glandular tissue of the breasts. The two areas of the physiological uptake will be giving the incidental findings especially related to the deserve special mention, namely, the thyroid gland and the gastrointestinal tract. The pattern of the uptake like the diffuse or focal uptake will be seen as in goitrous glands or thyroiditis. The closest differentials will be the malignancies or premalignant findings in as many as 33% of patients and should be further examined [12]. The Physiologic uptake in the bowel will be variable, resulting from the mild to the diffuse intense and focal uptake; more subtle in the caecum and rectosigmoid and also the patients undergoing treatment with metformin The exact cause of the intestinal uptake is not fully completely understood. The various factors which will be impacted are metabolically active mucosa, luminal contents, or glycolytic bacteria.

3. PET imaging applications

The clinical role of the correlative imaging will be used for various applications. And with the commercially available radiopharmaceuticals which are being used more commonly in various oncology [13], cardiology [14], neurology, and psychiatry [15, 16]. As discussed previously, the inner component of the PET/MR imaging design will be showing similarities of the MR head coil, PET detector ring, and MR magnet tunnel. Simultaneously acquired MR images, PET, and fused combined PET/MR images after intravenous injection of 370 MBq of FDG are shown. This tracer can be recorded for the 20 minutes at steady state till 2 hours. The earliest form of the image registration will be restricted to the various applications of the brain for the various brain tissues with the satisfactory model [17, 18]. Thus, the PET-CT is more useful for the neuroimaging applications and now one of the well-established imaging modalities. This also has the important role in the evaluation of the various central nervous system disorders like epilepsy, Alzheimer's and Parkinson's disease, head injury, and inoperable brain tumours [19–21].

The use of the various radiotracers for the assessment of the tumour metabolism and also the various physiological alteration involved in various diseases, and these are having significant impact on the PET/CT role as the emerging modality in the field of molecular imaging. The various oncological applications are being used for the evaluation of the [13, 22] various conditions in the central nervous system disorders, orthopaedic infections, and inflammatory disorders, and also for the evaluation and metastatic follow up of various pathologies.

PET imaging of radiolabelled nanoparticles has created lot of curiosity in the field of the molecular imaging. The size criteria's for the nanoparticles is related to the size range of the few to several hundred nanometres. Lot of advantages of the nanoparticles are there as the newer molecular imaging agents, which are not being limited by the ease of the physical properties and also for the surface functionalisation [23, 24]. Physically the nanoparticles will be having the larger surface area-to-volume ratio. These are capable of getting attached to the various targets which will be used as the targeting agents for the various diagnostic, and therapeutic purposes. These are the agents which will be providing the more specific binding receptor capacity with higher specificity and affinity which is more important for the more precise detection and the evaluation of the various disease markers. Another important property is that it will be having the longer half-life as compared to the free drug molecules resulting in the significantly enhanced bioavailability.

The important aspect is the important characteristics of the radioisotopes which are the imaging characteristics of isotopes; the decay half-life of the radioisotope; the isotope availability; and the reliability of the radiolabelling of the radioisotope. The lesser positron energy with the high branching ratio of β+ decay will be having the different characteristics for PET imaging. The use of the isotopes having the high positron energy will be travelling for the longer distance for the positron annihilating and will have the significant loss of the spatial resolution. The isotopes which are having the very low positron efficiency, will have the lower atoms undergoing the β+ decay as compared to the overall atoms which will be requiring the very long scan times and also the very noisy images [25].

The nanomaterial use in the biomedical engineering can be able to understand the better "absorption, distribution, metabolism, and excretion" (ADME) pattern for the materials which can strike the balance between the nanoparticle-induced benefits and also the long-term toxicity due to nanoparticle exposure [26–28]. As we all know that the PET imaging is having significant advantage of higher sensitivity and also the ability for the quantitative analysis of the whole-body imaging and due to this property the more precise biodistribution of nanoparticles can be done. Thus, the PET imaging can be able to monitor the various nanoparticles in the non-invasive manner. The labelling of the nanoparticles coordinating with the radiometal, and the chelator is more preferred option. There is also the alternative method of the evaluation.

3.1 Radiolabeled nanoparticles for molecular imaging

The nanoparticles are having the two important advantages. Different and multiple modalities can be useful for the various modalities to get integrated in the single nanoparticle platform. We all know at this point that every imaging modality is having the advantages and disadvantages. PET imaging resolution is very much sensitive upto the picomolar level and quantitative >1 mm which is very low. The magnetic resonance imaging (MRI) is having the submillimetre-level spatial resolution still having significantly low sensitivity. The use of the optical imaging is highly sensitive and easily accessible. But due to the scatter of light there is the limitation of the penetration depth and also the spatial resolution. With this the combination of the different imaging modalities will be complimentary to each other and will have better imaging quality. The nanomaterials due to its functionalization they can be prevented to get attacked by the immune system and can have longer circulation time. The multiple targeting ligands are being conjugated to a single nanoparticle which will be providing the significant enhanced receptor binding affinity by the polyvalency effect [29].

3.2 Special imaging techniques

This technique was described by Weissman and Carrau [30]. By this method of the puffing the cheeks, the oral vestibule is being filled with air, creating the negative contrast separating the buccal and labial mucosa from the gingival mucosa, and due to this both the mucosal surfaces can be evaluated separately. In this procedure the buccinators muscle, the pterygomandibular raphe, and the retromolar trigone are also seen better. The mucosal pliability is also being affected due to the trismus. So, during the FDG PET/CT acquisition if there is focal area of the uptake of FDG in the oral cavity then the use of the puffed-cheek maneuvere, should be done which will take around 4 minutes. Patient is asked to close the mouth and fully puff the cheeks while breathing through the nose during this 3- to 4-minute PET/CT acquisition. The puffed cheek scanning time is very short and can result into the more increased salivation and associated attenuation effects [31, 32]. This technique will lead to the better localisation and demonstration of the extent of a tumour of the oral cavity. Chang and colleagues [33] demonstrated that the puffed cheek maneuvere on FDG PET/CT is more useful for the evaluation of the oral cancers and their extent as seen in the FDG PET/CT. This study has shown that the localised or extended oral cancers of puffed cheek FDG PET/CT and conventional FDG PET/CT was 95.2% and 54.5%, respectively. FDG PET/CT delineated more oral cancers as compared to our routine conventional FDG PET/CT and also for the preoperative evaluation of the tumour thickness. The dental artefacts are significantly reduced by 70% in the puffed-cheek FDG PET/CT.

3.3 Open-mouth technique

Method is described by Henrot and colleagues [34]. In this technique the routine conventional whole-body FDG PET/CT done from the supraorbital margin to mid-thigh (**Figure 5**). After this the patient has to open the mouth. 50-mL syringe is put in between the teeth to for the correct immobilisation. The PET-CT is acquired during quiet respiration. PET/CT scan is again acquired from the orbitomeatal line to the clavicular fossa, with one field of view (15 cm, 3.5 minutes) and totally taking upto 3–4 minutes. The important indication of these is the evaluation of the tumour of the oral cavity and also the oropharynx which sometimes are difficult for the evaluation of the dental artefact. Cistaro and colleagues [32] have demonstrated that this technique is more useful in the evaluation of the oral carcinomas. With this the tumour localization, tumour extent, and surrounding structure involvement can be seen in this open-mouth view as compared with the closed mouth view.

Modified Valsalva maneuvere is used for the evaluation of the location and extent of a hypopharyngeal tumour as there will be the opposition of the mucosal surfaces and also for the evaluation of the nasopharynx when the pharyngeal recesses are collapsed. This maneuvere is done by asking the patient to utter the word "e" uniformly for at least 10 seconds and during this time the patient should hold breath for at least 10 seconds. It is advisable to instruct the patient before so that no artefacts can be seen. This technique is done from the hyoid bone to the trachea.

The phonation is indicated to differentiate between the true and false vocal cords which are needed to evaluate the precise location of the laryngeal tumour and its margins for the quiet respiration during the examination. With this the true vocal cords can be seen opposing and cannot be able to distinguish from each other as performed during the apnoea. Still, they can be abducted and not visible when the acquisition is performed during quiet respiration [34]. These techniques along with the modified Valsalva and phonation techniques are mostly used for the CT acquisition. The performing hybrid PET/CT along with this two maneuvere is difficult as the PET acquisition for one field of view requires a minimum time duration of 2–3 minutes The use of the spot and the various maneuvere will be leading to the better delineation of the hot spots [35]. Ter-Pogossian [1] showed that it will take 3 minutes to perform modified Valsalva or phonation technique for this period. There are many motion artefacts and due to this the coregistration of CT and PET images is very difficult.

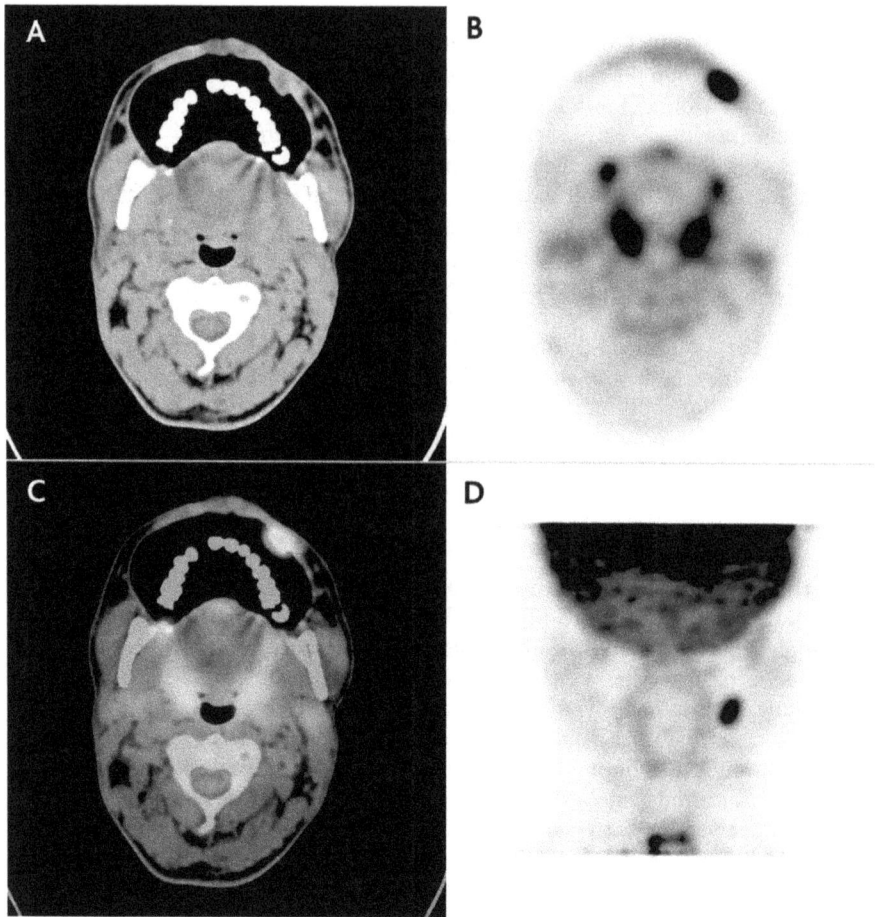

Figure 5.
This is the puff cheek technique which is very important for the evaluation of the small nodular lesion seen in the left buccal mucosa. CT image (A) showing nodule, (B and C) are the PET images and (C) image is the fused image showing nodular lesion with the significant uptake.

3.4 Optimization of patient preparation

The Optimization of scan protocol will lead to the decrease in the physiologic uptake of FDG in the head and neck region. The voluntary or involuntary tongue movement or sucking actions will cause in the significant increase in the pharyngeal muscles uptake [36]. The increased uptake in the base of the tongue and anterior part of the floor of the mouth is due to the increased uptake in the genioglossus muscle in the supine position due to its role of preventing the tongue to fall posteriorly and causing obstruction of the airway especially in the rest and also during the [37]. The other false uptake can be due to the activity post injection like talking and movement this is due to the increased laryngeal muscle activity [38]. The other areas of the uptake will be seen in the various muscles like lateral pterygoid, and masseter and this is also possible due to the long wait time [39]. Mid-morning is better time for the evaluation to prevent the supine position related FDG uptake in the muscles at the base of the tongue and anterior part of the mouth floor. FDG uptake in the brown fat and neck muscle can be difficult to differentiate between the supraclavicular lymph nodes and can be masked [40]. Ter-Pogossian [1] silent suggested not to have the liquid intake 30 minutes before the injection and also during the waiting time between FDG injection and whole-body scanning to avoid FDG uptake by the tongue and vocal muscles. Before the scan, all metal objects 7(eg, necklaces, earrings, and prosthesis) should be removed to prevent the metal attenuation artefacts. Cistaro and colleagues [32] showed the optimization of patient preparation in patients with HNC. With this technique there will be less FDG uptake in the muscles of base of tongue and floor of the mouth can be achieved. FDG, is not tumour-specific and various image interpretation pitfalls may occur because of false-positive and -negative causes of FDG uptake. The use of certain premedication, such as propranolol and diazepam, will result in the decrease physiologic FDG uptake in the brown fat and muscle.

3.5 Precision medicine

National Institutes of Health (NIH) has defined precision medicine as "an emerging approach for disease treatment and prevention that takes into account individual variability in genes, environment, and lifestyle for each person." This concept will be more useful for the doctors and researchers for evaluation of the various treatment options and other prevention aspects for the various diseases. Thus, leading to the various focus is on identifying different approach including the genetic, environmental, and lifestyle factors. The current therapy paradigm of "one-size-fits-all" approach, in which disease treatment and prevention strategies are developed.

3.6 Biomarker for precision diagnostics

A good and ideal biomarker for patient selection is very important for the evaluation of the novel therapeutic agent. Due to this there has to be companion diagnostic predictive markers, and these are being developed for the selection of the right patients. Tirapazamine (TPZ) is the benzothiazine series hypoxia-selective antitumor agent. PET/CT with fluorine-18-labelled fluoromisonidazole (18F-FMISO) or 18F fluoroazomycin arabinoside (FAZA) which is the hypoxic agent can be used with the TPZ [41, 42] as a diagnostic marker. PET/CT for the evaluation of the oestrogen receptor (ER) expression for the management and also with hormonal therapies for the various neuroendocrine tumour patients like the 68Ga DOTATATE PET/CT, before the initiation of the therapeutic management with 177LuDOTATATE [43]. The use of the 68GaPSMA PET/CT before therapy with 177Lu-PSMA therapy can also be evaluated [44]. Thus, there are more precise and the important new PET radiopharmaceuticals having the specific molecular targets, and also for the therapy along with these agents.

3.7 Tumour heterogeneity

The important aspect of the precision medicine use in the oncology is the tumour heterogeneity, but it is still challenging due to various reasons and most important one is the heterogenous presentation of the tumour. The heterogeneity of the tumour can be again sub classified as the (1) intertumoral heterogeneity: In this category the patient will be having different tumours or lesions which looks similar histologically but may be differing in the molecular variants as well as the malignant potential; (2) on contrary the intratumor heterogeneity: where the tumour will have the different functional capabilities in the tumour heterogeneity. The application of the spatial heterogeneity of subclones in a primary lesion or metastasis will be providing a bigger challenge for precision medicine as sequencing a portion of the tumour may miss important therapeutically relevant information. Lesions may be at locations who will get the tissue biopsy practically impossible. The end result of the clones can change with selective pressure from a targeted therapy leading to the of mutagenic activity of radiation and chemotherapy. Usually, the patient prognosis is poor when biomarkers found in the primary tumour, and metastatic lesions are varied. Thus, precision medicine will be requiring the different intratumor and intertumoral heterogeneity in the patient. The PET/CT is capable of the providing the different intratumor pattern of the heterogeneity along with the interpatient intertumoral heterogeneities. By this the evaluation of the whole-body can be done for the primary as well as metastatic lesion at one time. With the availability of the newer PET radiotracers, it will be possible for the evaluation of the intratumor and intertumoral heterogeneity. PET with 18F-FES can evaluate the regional ER expression [45] and this is having the advantage to overcome the different errors which will be arising the from disease heterogeneity. The use of the PET can also be able to measure the delivery and also the binding of oestrogen in vivo in correlation of the ER expression for the multiple tumour sites. The 18F-FES uptake in the tumour can be correlating with the ER expression corresponding to the various radioligand binding sites [45] the radiotracer uptake is directly related with the tamoxifen and aromatase inhibitor treatment [46–48]. Here the FES-PET is more important for the assessment of tumour heterogeneity of ER expression [49]. One of the recent study the role of the 18F-FES PET/CT can change the plan of the management upto the 48.5% of patients. For the detection of the ER status in the metastasis group (n 5 27), there will be significant increase in the 18F-FES PET/CT which has shown the significant increase in the metastatic lesions in 11 patients; absent in the 13 patients, and the rest of the 3 patients will be having both the 18F-FES positive and negative lesions. The 18F-FES PET/CT results has shown the better management plans in 16 patients (48.5%, 16/33) [50]. Another example is radiation therapy delivery which is significantly based on the heterogeneity of tumour hypoxia which is based on 18F-FMISO PET/CT [51]. The concentration of the 18F-FMISO in this gross tumour volume (GTV) is based on the hypoxia levels in the tumour. The 18F-FMISO PET/CT-guided intensity modulated radiotherapy (IMRT) for 10 patients in the diagnosed head and neck cancers which will be achieved 84 Gy to the GTV(h) and 70 Gy to the GTV, these can be done without exceeding the normal tissue tolerance levels. Investigators also attempted to deliver 105 Gy to the GTV(h) for 2 patients and were successful in 1, with normal tissue sparing.

3.8 Therapy assessment

The use of the various current therapy evaluations showing the anatomic changes, and these are the not sensitive biomarkers for the novel and targeted therapies. The basis here is the identification of the therapy resistance which needs to be evaluated early for the delivery of the precision medicine. The role of the PET/CT is important for the delivering precision medicine. Thus PET/CT is useful for the evaluation of the early therapy assessment along with the biology of the tumours or molecular subtypes, therapy selection, timing of early therapy assessment PET/CT, and for the performing PET/CT in a standardised manner.

4. Methionine

Methionine is the commonly used amino acid tracer, which is used in PET imaging of brain tumours, due to the low physiologic uptake of MET in brain. This is being used as it is very convenient for the radiochemical production, which will be allowing the rapid synthesis leading to the higher radiochemical yield [52]. The significant increased uptake of methionine is to be correlated with both cellular proliferation [53] and micro vessel count [54] in gliomas. Post injection, MET uptake in the brain is low and, in combination with high tumour uptake, leading to the very higher detection rate and also the good lesion delineation [55]. The normal biodistribution of the MET uptake is lower in the cerebral cortex, cerebellum, basal ganglia, and thalamus. Moderate amount of the accumulation is seen in pituitary and glandular system (parotid and salivary glands).

5. Choline

Prostate cancer is one of the most common malignancies in men and the incidence of prostate cancer increases directly with age. This tumour is showing the biologic behaviour, from a clinically silent, intraprostatic tumour to an aggressive malignancy, and resulting into the more sensitivity. Early identification is more helpful for the benefit of therapeutic decision-making [56, 57]. Prostate cancer cells are showing the significant increased phosphocholine levels along with the elevated turnover of the cell membrane phospholipid, namely phosphatidylcholine [58]. Choline imported into the cell which is again phosphorylated by choline kinase in the first step of the Kennedy cycle. The role of the choline kinase is more in the prostate cancers, and due to this the prostate cancers will have more carbon-11 choline concentrations in the cells [59]. The important characteristic of the CHO faster blood clearance (5 min) and also the significantly faster uptake in the prostate tissue (3–5 min), this will be resulting into early excretion in the urine. The longer half-life of fluorine-18 (110 min) allows transportation of 18F-fluorocholine to centres without a cyclotron [60], although 18F-choline has a higher urinary excretion than CHO [60].

6. Radiotracer advances

Due to the technical developments various new radiotracers are in pipeline for the more precise use of these in various cancers, which is capable of the evaluation of the cell proliferation, metastasis to different organs, hypoxia in various tumours, focussed receptor status, tumour antigen levels, and various therapeutic response.

[18]F-fluorothymidine (^{18}F-FLT) is being used as the cell proliferation marker which will be used for the better quantification of tumour growth and also for the metastatic work up and also for the treatment response evaluation [61, 62]. ^{18}F-Fluoromisonidazole (FMISO), is the important hypoxia biomarker for the evaluation of the degree of hypoxia in a tumour which can be used to see the aggressiveness of the tumour and also the response to management. This will introduce the various endothelial cells which are being activated by tumour-induced angiogenesis which can be used as an indicator of the local as well as the distant metastasis. The use of the ^{18}F-galacto-arginine-glycine-aspartic acid tripeptide, having the capacity to bind the primary tumours as well as the metastatic lesions. ^{68}Ga-PSMA, is being widely used as the radiotracer of choice with significant low FDG avidities. Thus, this PSMA is showing in the pathologies which are showing the low uptake. The use of the ^{18}F-Fluciclovine, is the analog used for the various pathologies. The use of the ^{18}F-Choline PET/CT is being used as the radiotracer of choice for the leptomeningeal metastasis detection.

The radiotracers which will be targeting the various hormone receptors and HER2 are the newer development, and they are having significantly increased efficacy. The use of the ^{18}F-16α-fluoroestradiol (FES) as an substrate of oestrogen receptors is seen widely and can be seen as the source of the ER expression and the pharmacodynamic marker in the ER-directed therapy [63]. The use of the ^{68}Ga-NOTA-RM26, is seen as the ER expression for the improvement in the sensitivity and specificity of breast cancer diagnosis which is seen as close to the 100 and 90.9%, respectively, in the proliferating phase of the menstruating cycles patients. Clinically HER2 status is determined by immunohistochemical or fluorescence *in situ* hybridization testing of biopsy samples. New PET tracers like the ^{89}Zr-trastuzumab and ^{89}Zr-pertuzumab are being used for the quantification of the HER2 expression of the primary tumour and metastases simultaneously which shows the promising results.

7. PET radiomics

Radiomics is the newer concept of using the various disease characteristics in which the various parameters/features can be taken in the region of interest like the mathematical algorithms. Non-invasive image-derived biomarkers are also generated from PET radiomics based on the pixels, their associated parameters, and their positions [64–66]. Since the MRI has significantly high sensitivity then the PET- and MRI combination will have better spectrum of features for the building of the predictive models.

8. Summary

The relevance of PET scan is the important aspect of the various techniques which can be used for the various clinical applications. The different protocols need to be set for the different conditions to have the better sensitivity of that particular pathologies. The use of different radiotracers also needs to be explained in detail for the evaluation on the lines of the precision medicine. The various clinical applications are based on the different techniques used as well as the different radiotracers used. The sensitivity of these are based on the using of the optimal parameters for the evaluation of the different tumours or the pathologies. Thus this chapter redefines the important aspects of the both techniques as well as the clinical applications.

Author details

Sikandar Shaikh
PET-CT and Radiology, Yashoda Hospitals, Hyderabad, India

*Address all correspondence to: idrsikandar@gmail.com

IntechOpen

References

[1] Ter-Pogossian MM, Raichle ME, Sobel BE. Positron emission tomography. Scientific American. 1980;**243**:170-181

[2] Hess S, Høilund-Carlsen PF, Alavi A. Historic images in nuclear medicine 1976: The first issue of clinical nuclear medicine and the first human FDG study. Clinical Nuclear Medicine. 2014;**39**:701-703

[3] Rich DA. A brief history of positron emission tomography. Journal of Nuclear Medicine Technology. 1997;**25**(1):4-11

[4] Alavi A, Reivich M. The conception of FDG-PET imaging. Seminars in Nuclear Medicine. 2002;**XXXII**(1):2-5

[5] Ido T, Wan CN, Casella V, et al. Labeled 2-deoxy-D-glucose analogs. Fluorine-18-labeled 2-deoxy-2-fluoro-D-glucose, 2-deoxy-2-fluoro-D-mannose, and C-14-2-deoxy-2-fluoro-D-glucose. Journal of Labelled Compounds and Radiopharmaceuticals. 1978;**14**:175-182

[6] Reivich M, Kuhl D, Wolf A, et al. The [18F]fluorodeoxyglucose method for the measurement of local cerebral glucose utilization in man. Circulation Research. 1979;**44**:127-137

[7] Karp JS, Surti S, Daube-Witherspoon ME, et al. Benefit of time-of-flight in PET: Experimental and clinical results. Journal of Nuclear Medicine. 2008;**49**(3):462-470

[8] Miller M, Griesmer J, Jordan D, et al. Initial characterization of a prototype digital photon counting PET system. Journal of Nuclear Medicine. 2014;**55**:658

[9] Wong WH, Li H, Zhang Y, et al. A high-resolution time-of-flight clinical PET detection system using the PMT-quadrant-sharing technology. Journal of Nuclear Medicine. 2014;**55**:657

[10] Bos R, van Der Hoeven JJ, van Der Wall E, et al. Biologic correlates of (18) fluorodeoxyglucose uptake in human breast cancer measured by positron emission tomography. Journal of Clinical Oncology. 2002;**20**:379-387

[11] Bertout JA, Patel SA, Simon MC. The impact of O_2 availability on human cancer. Nature Reviews. Cancer. 2008;**8**:967-975

[12] Shie P, Cardarelli R, Sprawls K, et al. Systematic review: Prevalence of malignant incidental thyroid nodules identified on fluorine-18 fluorodeoxyglucose positron emission tomography. Nuclear Medicine Communications. 2009;**30**(9):742-748

[13] Czernin J, Allen-Auerbach M, Schelbert HR. Improvements in cancer staging with PET/CT: Literature-based evidence as of September 2006. Journal of Nuclear Medicine. 2007;**48**:78S-88S

[14] Di Carli MF, Dorbala S, Meserve J, et al. Clinical myocardial perfusion PET/CT. Journal of Nuclear Medicine. 2007;**48**:783-793

[15] Costa DC, Pilowsky LS, Ell PJ. Nuclear medicine in neurology and psychiatry. Lancet. 1999;**354**:1107-1111

[16] Tatsch K, Ell PJ. PET and SPECT in common neuropsychiatric disease. Clinical Medicine. 2006;**6**:259-262

[17] Pelizzari CA, Chen GT, Spelbring DR, et al. Accurate three-dimensional registration of CT, PET, and/or MR images of the brain. Journal of Computer Assisted Tomography. 1989;**13**:20-26

[18] Woods RP, Mazziotta JC, Cherry SR. MRI-PET registration with automated

algorithm. Journal of Computer Assisted Tomography. 1993;**17**:536-546

[19] Gilman S. Imaging the brain. The New England Journal of Medicine. 1998;**338**:812-820

[20] Viergever MA, Maintz JB, Niessen WJ, et al. Registration, segmentation, and visualization of multimodal brain images. Computerized Medical Imaging and Graphics. 2001;**25**:147-151

[21] Muzik O, Chugani DC, Zou G, et al. Multimodality data integration in epilepsy. International Journal of Biomedical Imaging. 2007;**2007**:13963

[22] Bohnen NI, Djang DS, Herholz K, et al. Effectiveness and safety of 18F-FDG PET in the evaluation of dementia: A review of the recent literature. Journal of Nuclear Medicine. 2012;**53**(1):59-71

[23] Ma X, Zhao Y, Liang X-J. Theranostic nanoparticles engineered for clinic and pharmaceutics. Accounts of Chemical Research. 2011;**44**:1114-1122

[24] Cheon J, Lee J-H. Synergistically integrated nanoparticles as multimodal probes for nanobiotechnology. Accounts of Chemical Research. 2008; **41**:1630-1640

[25] Yoshida E, Tashima H, Inadama N, Nishikido F, Moriya T, et al. Intrinsic spatial resolution evaluation of the X'tal cube PET detector based on a 3D crystal block segmented by laser processing. Radiological Physics and Technology. 2013;**6**(1):21-27

[26] Soo Choi H, Liu W, Misra P, Tanaka E, Zimmer JP, Itty Ipe B, et al. Renal clearance of quantum dots. Nature Biotechnology. 2007; **25**:1165-1170

[27] Choi HS, Ashitate Y, Lee JH, Kim SH, Matsui A, Insin N, et al. Rapid translocation of nanoparticles from the lung airspaces to the body. Nature Biotechnology. 2010;**28**:1300-1303

[28] Wang B, He X, Zhang Z, Zhao Y, Feng W. Metabolism of nanomaterials in vivo: Blood circulation and organ clearance. Accounts of Chemical Research. 2012;**46**:761-769

[29] Starmans LW, Hummelink MA, Rossin R, Kneepkens E, Lamerichs R, Donato K, et al. 89Zr-and Fe-labeled polymeric micelles for dual modality PET and T1-weighted MR imaging. Advanced Healthcare Materials. 2015;**4**:2137-2145. DOI: 10.1002/ adhm.201500414

[30] Weissman JL, Carrau RL. "Puffed-cheek" CT improves evaluation of the oral cavity. American Journal of Neuroradiology. 2001;**22**:741-744

[31] Fatterpekar GM, Delman BN, Shroff MM, et al. Distension technique to improve computed tomographic evaluation of oral cavity lesions. Archives of Otolaryngology – Head & Neck Surgery. 2003;**129**:229-232

[32] Cistaro A, Palandri S, Balsamo V, et al. Assessment of a new 18F-FDG PET/CT protocol in the staging of oral cavity carcinomas. Journal of Nuclear Medicine Technology. 2011;**39**:7-13

[33] Chang CY, Yang BH, Lin KH, et al. Feasibility and incremental benefit of puffed-cheek 18F-FDG PET/CT on oral cancer patients. Clinical Nuclear Medicine. 2013;**38**(10):e374-e378

[34] Henrot P, Blum A, Toussaint B, et al. Dynamic maneuvers in local staging of head and neck malignancies with current imaging techniques: Principles and clinical applications. Radiographics. 2003;**23**(5):1201-1213

[35] Gupta T, Master Z, Kannan S, et al. Diagnostic performance of post-treatment FDG PET or FDG PET/CT imaging in head and neck cancer:

A systematic review and meta-analysis. European Journal of Nuclear Medicine and Molecular Imaging. 2011; **38**:2083-2095

[36] Kubota K. From tumor biology to clinical PET: A review of positron emission tomography (PET) in oncology. Annals of Nuclear Medicine. 2001;**15**:471-486

[37] Abouzied MM, Crawford ES, Nabi AN. 18F-FDG imaging: Pitfalls and artifacts. Journal of Nuclear Medicine Technology. 2005;**33**:145-155

[38] Kostakoglu L, Wong JCH, Barrington SF, et al. Speech-related visualization of laryngeal muscles with florine-18-FDG. Journal of Nuclear Medicine. 1996;**37**:1771-1773

[39] Rikimaru H, Kikuchi M, Itoh M, et al. Mapping energy metabolism in jaw and tongue muscles during chewing. Journal of Dental Research. 2001;**80**:1849-1853

[40] Kostakoglu L, Hardoff R, Mirtcheva R, et al. PET-CT fusion imaging in differentiating physiologic from pathologic FDG uptake. Radiographics. 2004;**24**:1411-1431

[41] Mitsudomi T, Morita S, Yatabe Y, et al. Gefitinib versus cisplatin plus docetaxel in patients with non-small-cell lung cancer harbouring mutations of the epidermal growth factor receptor (WJTOG3405): An open label, randomised phase 3 trial. The Lancet Oncology. 2010;**11**(2):121-128

[42] Zegers CM, van Elmpt W, Szardenings K, et al. Repeatability of hypoxia PET imaging using $[^{18}F]HX_4$ in lung and head and neck cancer patients: A prospective multicenter trial. European Journal of Nuclear Medicine and Molecular Imaging. 2015;**42**(12):1840-1849

[43] Strosberg J, Wolin E, Chasen B, et al. 177-Lu-dotatate significantly improves

progression-free survival in patients with midgut neuroendocrine tumours: Results of the phase III NETTER-1 trial. New England Journal of Medicine. 12 Jan 2017;**376**(2):125-135. DOI: 10.1056/NEJMoa1607427

[44] Baum RP, Kulkarni HR, Schuchardt C, et al. ^{177}Lu-labeled prostate-specific membrane antigen radioligand therapy of metastatic castration resistant prostate cancer: Safety and efficacy. Journal of Nuclear Medicine. 2016;**57**(7):1006-1013

[45] Mintun MA, Welch MJ, Siegel BA, et al. Breast cancer: PET imaging of estrogen receptors. Radiology. 1988;**169**(1):45-48

[46] Mortimer JE, Dehdashti F, Siegel BA, et al. Metabolic flare: Indicator of hormone responsiveness in advanced breast cancer. Journal of Clinical Oncology. 2001;**19**(11):2797-2803

[47] Mortimer JE, Dehdashti F, Siegel BA, et al. Positron emission tomography with 2-[18F]fluoro-2-deoxy-Dglucose and 16alpha-[18F]fluoro-17beta-estradiol in breast cancer: Correlation with estrogen receptor status and response to systemic therapy. Clinical Cancer Research. 1996;**2**(6):933-939

[48] Linden HM, Stekhova SA, Link JM, et al. Quantitative fluoroestradiol positron emission tomography imaging predicts response to endocrine treatment in breast cancer. Journal of Clinical Oncology. 2006;**24**(18):2793-2799

[49] Kurland BF, Peterson LM, Lee JH, et al. Between-patient and within-patient (site-to-site) variability in estrogen receptor binding, measured in vivo by 18Ffluoroestradiol PET. Journal of Nuclear Medicine. 2011;**52**(10):1541-1549

[50] Sun Y, Yang Z, Zhang Y, et al. The preliminary study of 16alpha-[18F]

fluoroestradiol PET/CT in assisting the individualized treatment decisions of breast cancer patients. PLoS One. 2015;**10**(1):e0116341

[51] Lee NY, Mechalakos JG, Nehmeh S, et al. Fluorine-18-labeledfluoromisonidazole positron emission and computed tomography-guided intensity-modulated radiotherapy for head and neck cancer: A feasibility study. International Journal of Radiation Oncology, Biology, Physics. 2008;**70**(1):2-13

[52] Langstrom B, Antoni G, Gullberg P, et al. Synthesis of L- and D-[methyl-11C]methionine. Journal of Nuclear Medicine. 1987;**28**:1037-1040

[53] Chung JK, Kim YK, Kim SK, et al. Usefulness of 11C-methionine PET in the evaluation of brain lesions that are hypo- or isometabolic on 18F-FDG PET. European Journal of Nuclear Medicine and Molecular Imaging. 2002;**29**:176-182

[54] Kracht LW, Friese M, Herholz K, et al. Methyl-[11C]-l-methionine uptake as measured by positron emission tomography correlates to microvessel density in patients with glioma. European Journal of Nuclear Medicine and Molecular Imaging. 2003;**30**:868-873

[55] Moulin-Romsee G, D'Hondt E, de Groot T, et al. Non-invasive grading of brain tumours using dynamic amino acid PET imaging: Does it work for 11C-methionine? European Journal of Nuclear Medicine and Molecular Imaging. 2007;**34**:2082-2087

[56] Albersen PC. A challenge to contemporary management of prostate cancer. Nature Clinical Practice Urology. 2009;**6**:12-13

[57] Avazpour I, Roslan RE, Bayat P, et al. Segmenting CT images of bronchogenic carcinoma with bone

metastases using PET intensity markers approach. Radiology and Oncology. 2009;**43**:180-186

[58] Ackerstaff E, Glunde K, Bhujwalla ZM. Choline phospholipid metabolism: A target in cancer cells? Journal of Cellular Biochemistry. 2003;**90**:525-533

[59] Farsad M, Schiavina R, Castelluci P, et al. Detection and localization of prostate cancer: Correlation of (11) C-choline PET/CT with histopathologic stepsection analysis. Journal of Nuclear Medicine. 2005;**46**:1642-1649

[60] Hara T, Kosaka N, Kishi H. PET imaging of prostate cancer using carbon-11-choline. Journal of Nuclear Medicine. 1998;**39**:990-995

[61] Smyczek-Gargya B, Fersis N, Dittmann H, Vogel U, Reischl G, Machulla HJ, et al. PET with [18F] fluorothymidine for imaging of primary breast cancer: A pilot study. European Journal of Nuclear Medicine and Molecular Imaging. 2004;**31**:720-724. DOI: 10.1007/s00259-004-1462-8

[62] Kenny L, Coombes RC, Vigushin DM, Al-Nahhas A, Shousha S, Aboagye EO. Imaging early changes in proliferation at 1 week post chemotherapy: A pilot study in breast cancer patients with 3'-deoxy-3'-[18F] fluorothymidine positron emission tomography. European Journal of Nuclear Medicine and Molecular Imaging. 2007;**34**:1339-1347. DOI: 10.1007/s00259-007-0379-4

[63] Zhang J, Mao F, Niu G, Peng L, Lang L, Li F, et al. Ga-BBN-RGD PET/ CT for GRPR and integrin $\alpha\beta$ imaging in patients with breast cancer. Theranostics. 2018;**8**:1121-1130. DOI: 10.7150/thno.22601

[64] Acar E, Turgut B, Yigit S, Kaya G. Comparison of the volumetric and radiomics findings of 18F-FDG PET/CT

images with immunohistochemical prognostic factors in local/locally advanced breast cancer. Nuclear Medicine Communications. 2019;**40**:764-772. DOI: 10.1097/MNM.0000000000001019

[65] Huang SY, Franc BL, Harnish RJ, Liu G, Mitra D, Copeland TP, et al. Exploration of PET and MRI radiomic features for decoding breast cancer phenotypes and prognosis. npj Breast Cancer. 2018;**4**:24. DOI: 10.1038/s41523-018-0078-2

[66] Moscoso A, Ruibal A, Dominguez-Prado I, Fernandez-Ferreiro A, Herranz M, Albaina L, et al. Texture analysis of high-resolution dedicated breast ^{18}F-FDG PET images correlates with immunohistochemical factors and subtype of breast cancer. European Journal of Nuclear Medicine and Molecular Imaging. 2018;**45**:196-206. DOI: 10.1007/s00259-017-3830-1

Chapter 5

Feature Extraction Methods for CT-Scan Images Using Image Processing

Anil K. Bharodiya

Abstract

Medical image processing covers various types of images such as tomography, mammography, radiography (X-Ray images), cardiogram, CT scan images etc. Once the CT scan image is captured, Doctors diagnose it to detect abnormal or normal condition of the captured of the patient's body. In the computerized image processing diagnosis, CT-scan image goes through sophisticated phases viz., acquisition, image enhancement, extraction of important features, Region of Interest (ROI) identification, result interpretation etc. Out of these phases, a feature extraction phase plays a vital role during automated/computerized image processing to detect ROI from CT-scan image. This phase performs scientific, mathematical and statistical operations/algorithms to identify features/characteristics from the CT-scan image to shrink image portion for diagnosis. In this chapter, I have presented an extensive review on "Feature Extraction" step of digital image processing based on CT-scan image of human being.

Keywords: medical images, CT-scan image, feature extraction, image processing, image diagnoses

1. Introduction

In recent medical revolution, Computer Aided Diseases Diagnoses (CADD) plays an important role. The basic aim of CADD is to detect diseases on the basis of human image as an input at low cost, better accuracy and patient's satisfaction. There are many bio-medical imaging technologies available such as Radiography, computed tomography (CT-Scan), electrocardiography (ECG), Ultrasound, magnetic resonance imaging (MRI), etc. All these medical imaging modalities are best suited depending on the type of diseases to be detected from human body [1, 2].

In the human body, e.g., arm, leg, scalp, etc., each and every bone plays an important role and function. **Figure 1(a)** shows human being's head CT-scan image; and **Figure 1(b)** shows human being's chest CT-scan image.

CADD system can be developed with the use of image processing. **Figure 2** depicts steps of digital image processing [2].

Figure 2 shows basic steps to perform digital image processing. Image acquisition is the process of obtaining a digitized image from a real world source using imaging devices e.g., camera, cell phone, CT-scan, MRI, ultrasound etc. Images which are acquired in the first step may be blurred, out of focus or noisy so, in the

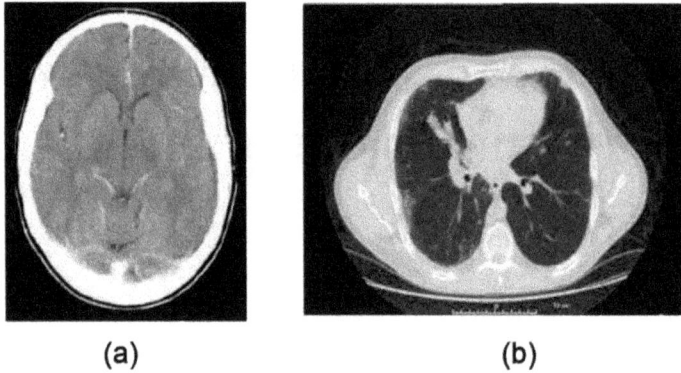

(a)   **(b)**

Figure 1.
(a) Head CT-scan image; and (b) chest CT-scan image. Courtesy: https://images.google.com/.

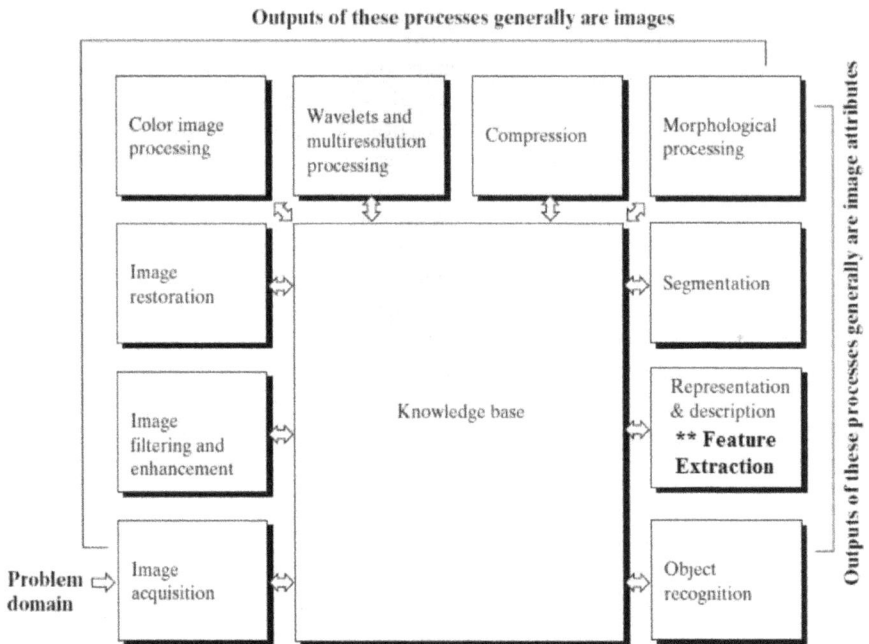

Figure 2.
Basic steps in digital image processing.

next step that is image filtering and enhancement which is used to improve the quality of image. This step includes various filtering and enhancement algorithms.

Image quality can also be improved with the use of Image restoration. The main difference between image enhancement and image restoration is that former is subjective and later is objective. Image restoration methods are based on mathematical/probabilistic models/algorithms of image degradation. While, Image enhancement methods are based on subjective liking of human preference during visualization [3]. The next step is Color Image Processing which deals with feature extraction on the basis of image color. Wavelet is the foundation for image resolution. This step focuses on use of wavelet to perform image resolution analysis. The next step is image compression. This step is used to decrease the size of image so that it can be stored in minimum space or can be transmitted even on low bandwidth channel. Morphological processing step includes tools for extracting image components that are useful in the step that is representation and description of image shape. The next step is image segmentation, it means dividing the image in constituent segments on the basis of boundary, similarity, color, shape etc.

Representation and description always follow the output of a segmentation step. The first option to be taken is whether to portray the data as a border or a complete region. When the focus is on external shape properties such as corners and inflections, boundary representation is appropriate. When the focus is on internal qualities such as texture or skeletal shape, regional representation is acceptable. A strategy for characterizing the data must also be defined in order to highlight features of interest. Description, also known as feature selection, is the process of selecting features that produce quantitative information of interest or are necessary for distinguishing one object class from another [3]. The last step is object recognition which deals with assigning the label to the object/information extracted during feature extraction step. Finally, the result is displayed in the form of data or image.

The aim of this chapter is to present an extensive research review on feature extraction sub-step of image processing cycle applied to human CT-scan images. The chapter is organized as follows: Section 2 gives a brief of different feature extraction techniques; Section 3 discusses work on CT-scan Image feature extraction; finally, the paper is concluded in Section 4.

2. Feature extraction techniques

Data/dimensionality reduction, which is performed by intelligently changing the image from the lowest level of pixel data into higher level representations, is a key component in image analysis. We can extract relevant information from these representations through a process known as feature extraction [4].

The ultimate aim in a large number of image processing applications is to extract important features from image data, from which a description, interpretation, or understanding of the scene can be provided by the machine [5].

As per Nixon and Aguado [6] feature extraction techniques are broadly classified into two categories that is low level feature extraction and high level feature extraction. Low-level features extraction deals with basic features that can be extracted automatically from an image without any shape information such as thresholding and edge detection.

Edge Detection: It highlights image contrast. Edge is generally boundary of the image objects where intensity of the pixel changes abruptly [6].

Thresholding: It chooses pixels within a specified range that have a specific value or arc. If the brightness level (or range) of an object is known, it can be used to locate it within a photograph. This implies that the brightness of the object must also be known [6].

Detecting image curvature (corner extraction): Curvature is normally defined by considering a parametric form of a planar curve. This technique is used to detect corner from the image [6].

Region/patch analysis: Collection of pixel is usually refers to region of the image. This technique is used to detect particular region on the basis of certain algorithm [6].

Hough transform: It defines an efficient implementation of template matching for binary templates. This technique is capable of extracting simple shapes such as lines and quadratic forms as well as arbitrary shapes [6].

Image motion detection: In the case of motion there is more than one image. If we have two images obtained at different times, the simplest way in which we can detect motion is by image differencing [6].

Histogram: The intensity histogram shows how individual brightness levels are occupied in an image; the image contrast is measured by the range of brightness levels [6].

Haar wavelets: Haar wavelets are binary basis functions. There is (theoretically) an infinite range of basis functions. Discrete signals can map better into collections of binary components rather than sinusoidal ones [6].

Texture extraction: Texture is an arrangement of pattern after certain interval in the image. Many techniques are used to extract texture from the image such as Local Binary Pattern (LBP), Fourier Transform, Co-occurrence matrices etc. [6, 7].

The above discussion provides brief overview of different techniques that can be used in digital image processing for the feature extraction from digital image. However, it is not an exhaustive discussion of the feature extraction techniques.

3. CT-scan image feature extraction

A feature extraction is a process through which region of interest (ROI) extracted for analyzing image. It includes modifying the image from the lower level of pixel data into higher level representations. From these higher level representations we can gather useful information; a process called feature extraction [8].

Ma and Wang [9] proposed a novel method to automatically detect the texts embedded in CT-scan Image. Authors have used Histogram of Oriented Gradients (HOG) as a statistical feature descriptor which reflects the distribution of oriented gradients in a selected region. Further, they have adopted AdaBoost classifier to separate the text regions from non-text regions. This method achieved 84% precision rate which is greater than edge base method (45%) and hybrid method (76%).

Shuqi et al. [10] proposed an algorithm to extract local features from mammographic image. In this paper, the SIFT algorithm is combined with the sliding window to extract the ROI region, that is, the breast region, and remove most of the background region. It follows the experimental process as Background de-noising, Using SIFT to extract the key point, Using the SVM and sliding window to detect the ROI position, Extract the features of the ROI region and Design BP neural network. The experimental results show that the accuracy of neural network classifier based on SIFT is 96.57%, which is 3.44% higher than that of traditional SVM classification accuracy.

Poomimadevi and Sulochana [11] presents an automated approach to detect tuberculosis using chest radiographs. The proposed approach basically includes three main steps such as Preprocessing, Registration and watershed segmentation. Lung region is extracted by using registration based segmentation methods. The accuracy of proposed segmentation and global thresholding is 59.8 and 59.4% respectively. While, the accuracy of active contour method is 34.4%. Joykutty et al. [12] also proposed a novel mechanism to detect tuberculosis in chest radiographs. The proposed method includes a three stage process of accurate detection of tuberculosis.

Barabas et al. [13] have developed a software namely Visualizer which allows the viewing of individual CT/MRI image slices, slice reconstruction in various projections, detailed analysis of slices and 3D reconstruction of desired object(s) as well as localization of various anatomical structures for further evaluation of parameters.

Chaudary and Sukhraj et al. [14] have worked on lung cancer detection from CT scan images using image processing steps such as pre-processing, segmentation and feature extraction. In this paper, authors have used MATLAB as image processing tool and concentrated on Area, Perimeter, Roundness and Eccentricity features of image.

Suzuki et al. [15] have used computer aided diagnostic scheme to detect abnormalities from Chest radiograph image of human beings using means of massive training artificial neural network.

Chen and Huang [16] presented an image feature extraction and fusion algorithm based on K-SVD, in order to better fuse CT and MRI images. The sliding window divides images into chunks in this technique. The column vectors are compiled into the dictionary. The K-singular value decomposition (K-SVD) approach is used to learn the redundant dictionary. The image feature fusion is then realized by solving the sparse coefficient matrix for each original picture and then combining sparse coefficient of nonzero members.

Ding et al. [17] have proposed a method based on the exploitation of features closely related to image inherent quality. Specifically, in the novel method, Sobel operator, log Gabor filter and local pattern analysis are employed for complementary representation of image quality. Finally, support vector regression is implemented for the synthesis of the multiple distortion indices and mapping the quantification into an objective quality score.

Litjens et al. [18] presented a survey on deep learning in CT-scan Image analysis. Authors have stated that feature extraction from CT-scan Image can also be done through efficient deep learning algorithm. Kaur and Jindal [19] have worked on OPEN CV Environment to extract features using SURF technique. They have emphasized on the feature extraction phase of content-based image retrieval (CBIR) [20] and concluded that SURF is efficient image processing technique in terms of detect ability, accuracy, rotation and execution time.

According to Hossein and Jacques [21], if prior shape and a straightened boundary image (SBI) based algorithm are applied on CT-scan Image segmentation then, feature extraction will be more easy. Using an adaptive thresholding technique, Oishila et al. [22] provided a tool that first segments the bone region of an input digital CT-scan Image from its surrounding flesh region and then generates the bone contour. It then undertakes unsupervised rectification of bone-contour discontinuities that may have been caused by segmentation mistakes, before detecting the presence of a fracture in the bone.

Seyyed et al. [23] has presented a novel feature which is the combination of shape and texture features. The feature extraction is started by edge and shape information of CT-scan Image then, Gabor filter is used to extract spectral texture features from shape images.

Ratnasari et al. [24] have concentrated on five statistical features like mean, standard deviation, skewness, kurtosis, and entropy to find out the CT-scan Image features for the development of computer applications for identification of lung tuberculosis (TB) disease and concluded that features extraction can be done effectively using combination of thresholding-based ROI template and PCA (Principle Component Analysis) methods.

Kazeminia et al. [25] proposed a novel method to eliminate the non-ROI data from bone CT-scan Images based on the histogram dispersion method. ROI is separated from the background and it is compressed with a lossless compression method. This method contains 3 steps such as Noise Reduction and Smoothing, ROI Boundary Detection and Compression.

Kumar and Bhatia [26] discussed different methods of feature extraction such as Diagonal based feature extraction technique, Fourier descriptor, Principal

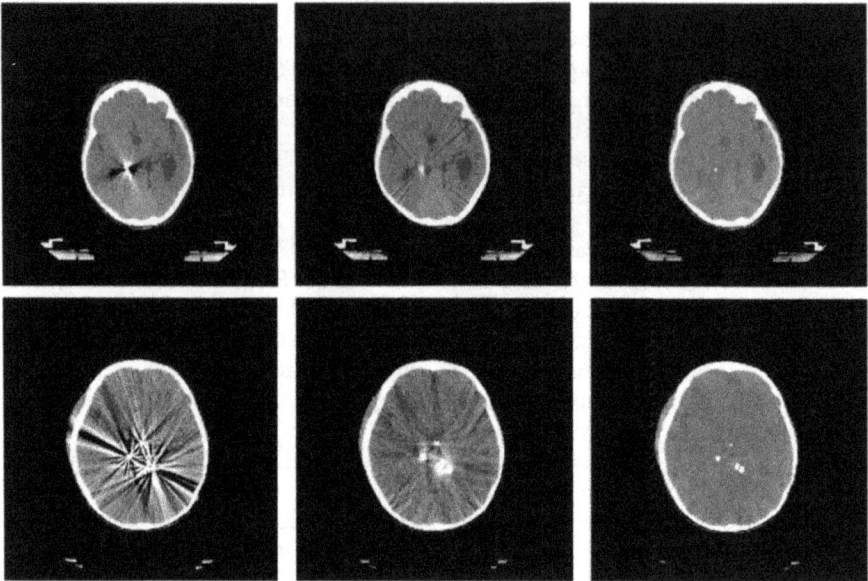

Figure 3.
Brain CT-scan image processing.

component analysis (PCA), Independent Component Analysis (ICA), Gabor filter, Fractal theory technique Shadow Features of character, Chain Code Histogram of Character Contour, Finding Intersection/Junctions, Sector approach for Feature Extraction, Extraction of distance and angle features, Extraction of occupancy and end points features, Transition feature and Zernike Moments.

As per Dubey et al. [27] edge detection techniques are also used for feature extraction. These techniques can be pewitt, sobel, Rober, Kirsch, Robinson, Marr-Hildreth, LoG, Canny etc.

Figure 3 shows image processing of human's brain CT-scan image. As per Kumar and Bhatia [26] and Dubey et al. [27], authors have implemented Gabor filter and edge detection technique to process the human brain CT-scan image in order to detect cancerous part of the brain. **Figure 3** is divided into 6 different sub-images as an output generated from the computerized digital image processing. In the first step original captured CT-scan image is fed to the system, image pre-processing and enhancement are conducted in the second step, edge detection using canny and prewitt method are done in the third step, fourth step focus on the Gabor filter in order to detect ROI, fifth step focuses on feature extraction using BLOB (binary large object) analysis and in the last that is step number 6 produces the final output image. Pseudocode of this process is given below:

```
Pseudocode: Human's brain CT-Scan image processing
READ CT-Scan image
CONVERT an inputted image into gray scale image(If RGB)
DO Pre-Processing and Image Enhancement
Do Edge detection using canny & prewitt methods
APPLY Gabor filter to detect ROI
DETECT features using BLOB analysis
DISPLAY processed CT-Scan image as an output
```

4. Conclusion and future attempts

X-Ray and CT-scan images is an important medical imaging component to detect bone related issues and diseases. Many researchers have shown their interest to work in the field of X-Ray image processing. The broad survey presented in the above section III proves that researchers have worked in features extraction from human being's X-Ray and CT-scan images. This research review is further useful for researchers to develop automatic application or decision support system to analyze human being's X-Ray and CT-scan images to detect bone related diseases such bone fracture identification, fatigue of knee joint, bone age assessment, lung module diagnoses, osteoporosis, arthritis, bone tumor, bone infection etc.

Author details

Anil K. Bharodiya
UCCC & SPBCBA & SDHG College of BCA & IT, Surat, Gujarat, India

*Address all correspondence to: anilbharodiya@gmail.com

References

[1] Bharodiya AK, Gonsai AM. Research review on human being's X-ray image analysis through image processing. In: Proceedings of National Conference on Sustainable Computing and Information Technology. Surat: SCET; 2017. pp. 38-42

[2] Bhowmik M, Ghoshal D, Bhowmik S. Automated medical image analyser. In: IEEE ICCSP 2015 Conference. New York: IEEE; 2015. pp. 0974-0978

[3] Gonzalez R, C., and Woods, R., E. Digital Image Processing. USA: PE & PH; 2008. pp. 1-34

[4] Mohamed MH, AbdeISamea MM. An efficient clustering based texture feature extraction for medical image. In: IEEE Proceedings of International Workshop on Data Mining and Artificial Intelligence, Bangladesh. New York: IEEE; 2008. pp. 88-93

[5] Jain AK. Fundamentals of Digital Image Processing. USA: PE & PH; 1989. pp. 342-425

[6] Nixon MS, Aguado AS. Feature Extraction & Image Processing for Computer Vision. Third ed. UK: Elsevier; 2012. pp. 137-212

[7] Rogers LF, Talianovic MS, Boles CA, et al. Grainger & Allison's Diagnostic Radiology: A Textbook of Medical Imaging. New York: Churchill Livingstone, Chap; 2008. p. 46

[8] Kodogiannisa VS, Boulougourab M, Wadgea E, Lygourasc N. The usage of soft-computing methodologies in interpreting capsule endoscopy. Elsevier Engineering Applications of Artificial Intelligence. 2007;**20**(4):539-553

[9] Ma Y, Wang Y. Text detection in medical images using local feature extraction and supervised learning. In: IEEE 12th International Conference On Fuzzy Systems and Knowledge Discovery (FSKD). New York: IEEE; 2015. pp. 953-958

[10] Shuqi C, Shen C, et al. Application of neural network based on SIFT local feature extraction in medical image classification. In: IEEE 2nd International Conference on Image, Vision and Computing. New York: IEEE; 2017. pp. 92-97

[11] Poomimadevi CS, Sulochana HC. Automatic detection of pulmonary tuberculosis using image processing techniques. In: IEEE WiSPNET Conference. New York: IEEE; 2016. pp. 798-802

[12] Joykutty B, Satheeshkumar KG, Samuvel B. Automatic tuberculosis detection using adaptive Thresholding in chest radiographs. In: IEEE International Conference on Emerging Technological Trends. New York: IEEE; 2016

[13] Barabas J, Capka M, Babusiak B, et al. Analysis, 3D reconstruction and anatomical feature extraction from medical images. In: IEEE International Conference on Biomedical Engineering and Biotechnology. New York: IEEE; 2012. pp. 731-735

[14] Chaudhary A, Sukhraj SS. Lung cancer detection on CT images by using image processing. In: IEEE International Conference on Computing Sciences. New York: IEEE; 2012. pp. 142-146

[15] Suzuki K et al. False-positive reduction in computer-aided diagnostic scheme for detecting nodules in chest radiographs by means of massive training artificial neural network. Academic Radiology. 2005;**12**(2): 191-201

[16] Chen H, Huang ZH. Medical Image Feature Extraction and Fusion

Algorithm Based on K-SVD. In: IEEE Ninth International Conference on P2P, Parallel, Grid, Cloud and Internet Computing. New York: IEEE; 2014. pp. 333-337

[17] Ding Y, Zhao Y, Zhao X. Image quality assessment based on multi-feature extraction and synthesis with support vector regression. Elsevier Signal Processing: Image Communication. 2017;**54**:81-92

[18] Litjens G, Kooi T, Babak EB, et al. A survey on deep learning in medical image analysis. Elsevier Medical Image Analysis. 2017;**42**:60-88

[19] Kaur B, Jindal S. An implementation of feature extraction over medical images on OPEN CV environment. In: IEEE International Conference on Devices, Circuits &Communications. New York: IEEE; 2014

[20] Swati VS, Vrushali GN. Design of Feature Extraction in content based image retrieval (CBIR) using color and texture. International Journal of Computer Science & Informatics. 2011;**I**(II):57-61

[21] Hossein MM, Jacques AD. Enhanced X-ray image segmentation method using prior shape. IET Computer Vision. 2017;**11**(2):145-152

[22] Oishila B, Arindam B, Bhargab BB. Long-bone fracture detection in digital X-ray images based on digital-geometric techniques. Elsevier Computer Methods and programs in Biomedicine. 2016;**123**:2-14

[23] Seyyed MM, Mohammad SH, et al. Novel shape texture feature extraction for medical X-ray image classification. International Journal of Innovative Computing, Information and Control. 2012;**8**(1-B):659-673

[24] Ratnasari NR, Adhi S, Indah S, et al. Thoracic X-ray features extraction using thresholding-based ROI template and PCA-based features selection for lung TB classification purposes. In: IEEE 3rd International Conference on Instrumentation, Communications, Information Technology, and Biomedical Engineering (ICICI-BME). New York: IEEE; 2013. pp. 65-69

[25] Kazeminia N, Karimi SM, Soroushmehr R, et al. Region of interest extraction for lossless compression of bone X-ray images. In: 37th Annual International Conference of the IEEE Engineering in Medicine and Biology Society (EMBC). New York: IEEE; 2015. pp. 3061-3064

[26] Kumar G, Bhatia PK. A detailed review of feature extraction in image processing systems. Fourth International Conference on Advanced Computing & Communication Technologies. 2014;**2014**:5-12. DOI: 10.1109/ACCT.2014.74

[27] Dubey P, Dubey PK, Changlani S. A hybrid technique for digital image edge detection by combining second order derivative techniques log and canny. In: 2nd International Conference on Data, Engineering and Applications (IDEA). New York: IEEE; 2020. pp. 1-6. DOI: 10.1109/IDEA49133.2020.9170672

www.ingramcontent.com/pod-product-compliance
Lightning Source LLC
Chambersburg PA
CBHW081242190326
41458CB00016B/5880